Prai:

"Scott Damian writes with great insight into the daily struggles of a person who stutters. Whether it is answering the telephone, talking in front of the class, or ordering in a restaurant, these are everyday challenges for those who stutter. I believe this book can and will make a difference in the lives of the many people who struggle with this distressing disorder."
~ **Jane Fraser**, President, The Stuttering Foundation

"So Inspiring! Goes to the core of what human perseverance is all about!"
~ **Heather Provost**, Broadway Producer for *Reasons To Be Pretty*, and *[title of show]*

"As a writer and user of many voices, I love Damian's *Voice*. It's a terrific read!"
~ **James Arnold Taylor**, voice over actor – Obi Wan Kenobi: *Clone Wars*, Fred Flinstone, Johnny Test, Ratchet: *Ratchet and Clank*

"Damian's heroic journey mirrors the journey we must all take."
~ **Keri Tombazian**, Voice over Actress/Radio Host 94.7 The Wave

SCOTT DAMIAN

V-V-VOICE

a stutterer's odyssey

Behler
PUBLICATIONS
USA

Behler Publications

Voice: A Stutterer's Odyssey
A Behler Publications Book

Copyright © 2014 by Scott Damian
Cover design by Yvonne Parks - www.pearcreative.ca.
Cover photo by Aaron Mendez

Library of Congress Cataloging-in-Publication Data

Damian, Scott.
  Voice : a stutterer's odyssey / by Scott Damian.
    pages cm
  ISBN 978-1-933016-84-9 (pbk.) -- ISBN 1-933016-84-1 (pbk.) -- ISBN 978-1-933016-83-2 (ebook) 1. Damian, Scott--Health. 2. Stutterers--Biography. 3. Stutterers--Rehabilitation. 4. Stuttering--Psychological aspects. I. Title.
  RC424.D238 2013
  616.85'54--dc23
                                2013024082

FIRST PRINTING

ISBN 13: 9781933016-84-9
e-book ISBN 9781933016-83-2

Published by Behler Publications, LLC
North Fayette, PA
www.behlerpublications.com

Manufactured in the United States of America

For Nettie
For Lynda and Raymond
For all those who yearn to speak...this is for you.

Table of Contents

Prologue
Not So Long Ago, Not So Far Away

The *Star Wars* theme pulses through the speakers on stage. Standing in the wings, I wait for my cue. Through the backstage intercom, I hear the tinny voice of the stage manager, "And we're a go, Scott."

The music rises, and it's show time!

I clomp up the iron ramp for the hundredth time, my futuristic robe flowing around my torso, knee high brown boots emphasizing my elongated stride, while the clipped light saber sways back and forth on my hip. Making my way onto the Tomorrowland stage at Disneyland, I feel the Southern California sun radiating down. My robe traps the sweltering heat, but the humidity doesn't discourage me from my job.

Taking center stage, I reach down, unfasten my light saber, and perform a few wushu moves. I strike a badass pose and applause explodes from the crowd. I'm doing what I do best. I am an actor, and I am a Jedi—at least for today.

Surrounding me is an array of faces, some dark and some light. All of them wear the same enthusiastic expression. Through my microphone headset, I ask the audience what most of them have come to hear: "WHO WANTS TO BE A JEDI KNIGHT?"

Excited hands dart high in the air—small hands, big hands, young hands, old·hands. Everybody wants to be part of something bigger. My eyes scan the audience; I catch sight of an adrenalized child in the front row wearing a Yoda T-shirt. He bounces up and down as if he's cracked out on sugar. Mickey Mouse ears lean to one side on his head, while he waves his hand in the air and moans, "OOOOOHHHH" through his puckered lips.

His fervor makes me smile. As hundreds of hands shake and swish around me, I can't keep my eyes off of him. There's something about this child. What is it? *Pick him!*

I descend from the stage and reach out to the boy. In my deep Jedi cadence, I ask, "You, young Padawan, do you wish to become a Jedi knight?"

The boy's eyes open wide and shine with excitement. He smiles, and I see sticky pink goo outlining his mouth. The boy looks up at his mother and she nods, giving him her blessing. I take hold of his hand and lead him to the stage.

He squeezes my hand hard with purpose, transferring the tacky goo of his fingers to mine. Either way, I don't mind. I'm completely taken by the innocence of his "I-don't-care-how-I-look" appearance. I really dig this kid.

I lead him to center stage, kneel down in front of him and ask him his age. As he raises five fingers, I hear a few "ahhhh's" from the audience.

"My little one, what is your name?"

He opens his mouth, shakes slightly and stomps his feet, "B-B-B-B…" He stops and tries again. "B-B-B…"

His face lowers as he fiddles with his fingers. I push away slightly from him, my head tilts, and my brow crinkles. A rush of heat fills me, and I'm almost overwhelmed by a deep, heart-wrenching reaction to his stammer. *It can't be THAT*, I tell myself.

The boy's mother calls out, "His name is Ben."

"Oh, like Ben Kenobi!" I exclaim. "Then you must be brave."

I wink, and a radiant smile flashes across the boy's face. To my relief, the audience applauds. "Now, young Ben, I will show you a combination that will help you defeat the dark side. Are you ready?"

His hands come together as his fingers tighten around one another. His mouth begins to open, and I know he's about to say something, when, suddenly, his eyes roll back as his body quivers again. *Oh, God, I know this look.*

"D-D-D-D-o y-y-y-you th-th-th-think I-I-I-I c-c-c-c-can m-m-m-m-meet Y-Y-Y-Yod-d-d-da?" the boy struggles to ask.

His stammer echoes through my microphone. The audience is silent, still. No one moves. Ben looks around, confused as all eyes focus on him. A few boys giggle from the audience. Ben looks away from the crowd and shakes his head. A frown arches on his face, and his chin begins to tremble.

No, Ben, don't give into it, I think to myself, as I remain frozen. Even though I try, I can't move. Suddenly, I realize that I don't want to finish this show. The Jedi is gone. The actor is gone. Now, it's only me standing here, staring at this fragile creature in front of me.

I want to take Ben in my arms and hold him tightly, protect him, and tell him he's not a freak. I want him to ignore the unrelenting jeers and shun the judging eyes. I want him to realize that these people will never understand him.

I don't want to whisk Ben away to a time long ago, in a galaxy far, far away. All I want to do is take him to another time, not so long ago, not so far away, where another frail boy encountered brokenness and defeat, struggle and victory, and ultimately stepped onto his own Yellow Brick Road and began his journey to find his voice.

My voice.

1 Don't Answer the Door

When you are a mother, you are never really alone in your thoughts. A mother always has to think twice, once for herself and once for her child."
— *Sophia Loren*

Memories. I watch as they cascade through my mind, like melting ice released after having been frozen for years. There was a time I chose to fast-forward through them or simply push them aside—too painful to observe, yet too abundant to ignore.

Now, my eyes are closed, but the eyes of my heart remain wide open. When did it all start, Ben? When was the beginning?

Recalling the first time I stuttered is like trying to pinpoint the first time I crawled or took my first steps. I know it happened, I just can't remember the exact moment it started. All I know is that my stuttering came like a wolf in sheep's clothing, cloaked in normalcy. At first, my stammering resembled the regular verbal patterns of any two-year old. Later, as I graduated from gibberish, I began uttering fragmented words like, "m-m-milk," or "gi-gi-give." They sounded charming at first, just normal hiccups in the fluency of any child.

When I expressed myself in those early years, a loving smile from Momma would follow, or a pat on the head from Pop. "Good job," they would remark, presuming I was just a typical kid searching for his audible rhythm. I still remember their affirming praises with gratitude, for they instilled in me my first taste of pride in my maturing vocal abilities.

When I turned four, my speech grew worse, and my impediment became more apparent. The clicking consonants and sputtering vowels increased. Soon, I began to sense that something damaged lived within me, within my mouth, yet I continued to express myself as I clung to the euphoria that accompanies childhood…until that memorable day.

Damn, it was so long ago, Ben.

It was March 1978, and I hunched over Luke Skywalker and Darth Vader while the battle between good and evil unfolded in front of me. CLACK! The pounding of action figures slapped together, echoing throughout the entranceway of my house — the small, one story home that Momma and Pop purchased three years after their 1969 marriage.

"Frugal" was the word my family lived by. My parents weren't born with silver spoons in their mouths; Pop worked under cars and Momma worked behind a desk for an accounting firm. They had five mouths to feed, which included Momma Nettie, our no-nonsense great-grandmother who lived in the corner room of our house. For me, frugality was the norm. I craved mac 'n cheese on a daily basis. To my young taste buds, it tasted like a grand feast. The Spiderman tank top I sported felt more like a tuxedo than a K-Mart special. And my heart fluttered with glee whenever I whirled around my small collection of toys in my private solar system.

A crashing sound shrilled from the back of my throat as the figures pummeled each other again. Tossing Darth Vader onto the linoleum, I held Luke Skywalker high into the air. Once again, he had triumphed. Good guys always won. I hummed an off-pitch song.

GLING, GLONG!

My oral symphony was short–lived by the interruption of a sound I had heard so many times before, yet never this close. Jumping out of my skin, I faced the door, my heart pounding like a freight train. Someone always safeguarded my interactions with ringing phones, but never with the doorbell. Mustering up some courage, I weighed my options: Should I call for someone to open the door, or just answer it?

Just open it. You're a big boy now, I finally convinced myself. As I yanked on the latch, Momma had already whisked past me, knocked my hand to the side, and pushed on the lock. "I got it, baby," she said with an air of urgency. The door flung open, stopping just inches from me. As I stepped back, facing the door, I listened to the exchange on the other side.

"Hello," said a deep voice. "Just sign here, ma'am."

I heard a pen scribbling on paper. "Thank you so much," Momma said.

My head wobbled back and forth, longing to peek around the corner of the door and see who stood on our front porch, but I'd been taught to let the adults speak. In my household, we weren't allowed to interrupt or listen in on "grown-up" conversations.

"Excuse us, but we're talking, could you go to your room?" was a common request in the house. Eavesdropping equated a sin, or so it seemed.

Closing the door behind her and placing the parcel to the side, Momma leaned on the door. She sighed, looking out of sorts, and I wondered what could possibly be wrong with her. In the early months of that year, Momma's responses were becoming more abrasive regarding my interaction with the outside world. She would push me away and answer the phone before my hands reached up to the ringing receiver, or speak for me when a McDonald's employee asked if I wanted a toy with my Happy Meal.

It wasn't the same with my older brother, though. Momma regularly let him speak for himself or answer the phone without supervision. As a testament to my independence, I hoped that maybe one day my parents would let me open the door or pick up the phone when I got older.

Noticing my fretful expression, Momma sank down beside me. "Don't answer the door, okay? You can't be doing things like that. Not now, anyway. Let one of us answer it. Do you understand?"

"Y-Y-Y-Y-e-e-es, m-m-m-ma'am," I replied.

Her eyes welled up with tears as she turned her head, averting eye contact with me. Biting her lip, she looked miserable, and I flung my body forward to embrace her. With my mind reeling, I suddenly realized that my unusual speech patterns were directly linked to Momma's abrupt breakdown.

Looking back now, I know my parents tried to put on a brave face when it came to my early stages of stuttering. They were trying to shield me from my disability — at least until they found a solution. Momma would force a grin as she patted my arm, urging me to calm down when I spoke. Pop would repeat, in his Guatemalan accent, "Take your time, you'll outgrow it." To hear their child struggle with words must have been heart wrenching, but their poker faces told a different tale.

These responses were a far cry from their jovial praises two years earlier, but I suspect my folks knew there was a long, rocky road ahead of me. It was their job to protect me, and they did the best they could to keep my confidence up and my sanity intact.

Besides, there was no way I could comprehend the severity of my speech impediment. Since I didn't leave my house unattended, I had never been exposed to outsiders looking at me weirdly, or hear rude remarks flung my way. That would come later. Yet, the more I expressed myself, the more I knew there was a monster in the closet who didn't have a name as of yet.

No, at this juncture in my life, my family spoke for me and thus, passively isolated me. On the other hand, thanks to my parents' protection, my early childhood was a joyful experience. Home was a secured haven where my fantasies ran amuck in an endless playground. The living room was transformed into the hull of a spaceship. The backyard monkey swings had morphed into a dangerous jungle, where I swung and climbed, hoping to save an imaginary damsel in distress. My room became a cave where dragons were slain, as I personified the classic knight in shining armor.

Everything in my little world seemed in check, until that day when I embraced Momma as reality reared its ugly head, giving me my first glimpse of a dubious future. I leaned my cheek on her shoulder and felt Momma's body tremble. *Is she crying?* I wondered. I didn't want to look at her, and I didn't want to push away, either. All I wanted Momma to feel was the weight of my body.

Don't worry, Momma, Pop is right. I'll outgrow it — whatever "it" might be.

But what if Pop was mistaken? What if I didn't outgrow whatever this was? What if Momma kept getting upset whenever I spoke? What would I do then?

2 It Ain't Easy Being Green

"Consider how much more you often suffer from your anger and grief, than from those very things for which you are angry and grieved."
—Marcus Antonius

I developed a habit after the doorbell incident. Obsessively, I started to examine my family's phonetic patterns, observing their lips as they moved when speaking, and comparing my hesitant voice to their fluency. Soon, I realized that my physical gyrations and long, drawn-out, clicking consonants were an anomaly in a house of articulated voices. I began to feel disconnected from my family, and more connected to whatever beast my protectors were trying to conceal from me.

But before I allowed this newfound revelation to affect my self-esteem, days whisked by and normal day-to-day distractions took over—my action figures fought one another, goblins chased me through the house, and I happily squirted mounds of ketchup on my mac 'n cheese. My daily routines were unspoiled diversions from my pessimistic thoughts. All seemed right in my simple world again, until another harrowing event unfolded unexpectedly.

As on every Friday afternoon, the house belonged to Momma Nettie and me. Momma and Pop were working, and my brother attended school. Alone in the living room—as usual—I propelled my Hulk action figure from the couch to the opposite chair of the room, as if he'd leapt over a chasm in the Grand Canyon.

I glanced up at the clock. It was almost three in the afternoon. In just a few minutes, Momma Nettie would brew her chicory coffee and butter some toast. I'd dunk my buttery deliciousness into the thick java while we watched Bob Barker call for a contestant to "come on down" on *The Price Is Right*. The tang of that coffee made me feel like a grown-up, and I loved Momma Nettie for giving me a taste of maturity.

I knocked on her bathroom door. "I-I-It's B-B-B-Bob B-B-Barker t-time!" She said she'd be out of the bathtub in just a few minutes. Most evenings, Momma Nettie pampered herself with a relaxing bubble bath and a few drags from her cigarettes. But this particular afternoon, she decided to partake in her nightly ritual during the daytime. She had bingo that night, and come hell or high water, she wasn't going to pass up one of her favorite games. If anyone in our house deserved some pampering and a game of high-stakes bingo, it was my seventy-year-old great-grandmother.

Nettie Bongard always put family first. Almost singlehandedly, she raised two children of her own, survived a divorce, put my Momma through school, and helped my parents raise my brother and I. Selfishness didn't exit in her daily mantra. Our great-grandmother gave her all to us. Representing the archetypal Cinderella, Momma Nettie did the laundry, the ironing, the cooking, and lavished us with love and discipline during those precious times before the cancer took over. I can still hear her constant discipline reverberating in my head thirty-four years later, "Scrub those teeth really good. They're the only ones you got!" "Clean behind your ears. That's where the funk is!" "Wipe your hiney. You don't want to stain your underwear." For me, her old-school lessons are still laced with poetry and practicality.

Continuing my adventures with The Hulk, and awaiting Momma Nettie's exodus from the bathroom, I was startled by the sudden clanging of the phone on the kitchen wall. The incessant ringing brought forth an unequaled paranoia. I clutched The Hulk like a crucifix as Momma's instructions echoed in my head, "Let one of us answer it."

Walking around in a circle and humming to myself, I tried to drown out the constant ringing. I heard Momma Nettie bellow out from the bathroom, "Can someone please answer that phone?"

The word "someone" grabbed my attention. Perhaps Momma Nettie knew something I didn't, and perhaps someone had come home without my knowledge. I zipped into every room of our house, hoping to find a familiar face, but all I found were empty beds and unruffled sheets. Momma Nettie probably wasn't thinking clearly, and she must have thought someone was home to protect me from the phone. Someone always did, but not on this day. Not this time.

The jangling from the phone persisted.

"Please, someone answer the damn phone???" Momma Nettie grumbled.

As I crept up to the kitchen phone, an idea hit me like a ton of bricks. I decided I was going to answer it. Glancing at my Hulk figure, I felt a burst of inspiration. I studied his rippled forearms, enormous muscles, and his gritted teeth.

Hulk was furious, menacing, and always ready to do battle. If he was so fearless, why couldn't I be, too? I picked up the receiver and, placing it to my ear, I opened my mouth. The word was there in my head, in neon colors—H. E. L. L.O.

My legs went numb. The tension tightened in my throat. Like static from a radio, a hard, crackling sound emitted from my mouth, "He-He-He…" I actually said something. At least, I'd said something. Now I had to push forward and keep the word flowing from my mind and out through my mouth.

"Hello?" inquired the male voice from the other end.

My staccato increased, "He-He-He-He-He-He…"

"Is anybody there?" the man asked.

"He-He-He-He-He-He…"

Then, Momma Nettie called out, "WHO'S ON THE PHONE?"

"Look, is someone there? I can hear you," said the impatient voice.

"He-He-He-He-He…"

"WHO IS IT?" Momma Nettie yelled.

There were too many sounds, too much to contend with. I felt as if I was being pulled in eighty different directions. My hand slammed on the countertop.

"This is rude," said the man on the other end. "Is this some kind of a joke?"

I pushed the word out harder, but it kept sticking in my mouth like chewed up bubble gum. "He-He-He-He-He…" My foot stomped on the floor, trying to kick-start the word. Momma was right, I should have let someone else answer it.

"Well, this is just rude. You're rude, you freak!" said the frustrated voice.

SLAM!

A clipping sound snapped in my ear. He had hung up. My head swirled, blurring everything around me as the man's words repeated in my ears, beating in my head senselessly: *"I can hear you!" "This is rude!" "You freak!"*

I dropped the receiver and heard it crack on the tiled floor. Something unimaginable slowly erupted from me—a burning, quaking sensation that made its way through my body. The hairs on my head stood up. My teeth clamped into a vise.

I saw the caller's face illuminate before me, and imagined him on the other end of the phone—slick black hair, sunken eyes, high cheekbones, a tailored suit, and a smarmy look to his face as red horns protruded out of his head. He didn't know my condition. He didn't know how it felt. He didn't have a clue.

As a boy growing up in a protected world, shame had never entered my soul. Ashamed of whom I was, ashamed of the whirring sounds that erupted from my mouth, ashamed for being misunderstood. At this poignant moment, I knew exactly why my family was trying to protect me. In an instant, the fairytales slipped away, vaporizing into thin air. *You're rude, you freak.*

I rushed to my bedroom, slammed the door shut, and stood perfectly still. I didn't know what to do with myself. I looked up and there, on a poster above my bunk bed, an illustration of The Hulk stared down at me. As he slammed through a brick wall with fury, I heard him telling me, *"Let it out! You can turn green, too!"*

Something clicked in my head and I leaned forward with clenched fists. When I hit the hollow wall in front of me, I reeled, then came back and hit it again, and again, and again. The hole got bigger. The dense layer of wall cracked around the edges while pieces of thin plaster went everywhere. I couldn't even feel my knuckles. All I could feel was the embarrassment, the wrath, and the loneliness.

I'm a freak, I'm a freak, I'm a freak, I silently repeated to myself, as each punch grew stronger.

Heavy footsteps thumped outside of my bedroom door, and then, without warning, Momma Nettie barged into the room—a white robe tied firmly around her drenched body.

"Baby!" she cried, jumping toward me and wrapping her arms around my waist. "Stop!"

We fell to the floor, but my rage continued as I tried to break away from her embrace. Like a wounded animal, I emitted a deep, guttural growl. But even though I kicked and punched the air, Momma Nettie's hold on me was firm as she pleaded, "Calm down, baby, please calm down."

Her voice trembled, and I felt her body quiver as she tried to restrain me. Then, like waking up from a nightmare, my senses took over and I stopped swinging my arms and legs. I wanted Momma Nettie to be safe, hopefully unscathed from my tantrum. Instead, as I looked up, I saw a frightened reaction shining from her blue eyes—a look I had never seen before. Blood had smeared on her white robe and, at first, I thought the blood belonged to Momma Nettie. But then I glanced at my fists. My knuckles were torn, slightly split from the violent outburst.

"I'm sorry, baby. I didn't know you had to answer the phone. I didn't." Momma Nettie apologized, undoubtedly distraught.

I peered up at The Hulk poster. He was still gawking down at me. In an instant I knew that was me. That was what I had become, a nightmarish fiend who walked out of a freak show. The Hulk and I were both monsters.

Breaking free from Momma Nettie's grip, I crawled to the farthest corner and yelled, "D-D-Don't c-c-c-come n-n-near m-m-m-m-me!"

The thought of hurting one of the most precious women in my life added more humiliation to my already distraught state. Momma Nettie froze, staring at me as if I had morphed into a stranger. And I had, not only to her, but to me as well. The fist was easy. The voice was impossible. The rage would continue.

3 You Won't Like Me When I'm Angry

"To be great is to be misunderstood."
— *Ralph Waldo Emerson*

As the weeks went by, the walls around the house resembled Swiss cheese. Little fist-sized grooves had ripped through the thin wallpaper, along with cracks and divots on the doors—all evidence of the rage that ignited when anything sputtered out of my mouth.

My fists knew no boundaries when the temper erupted. My arms and knuckles seemed possessed, as if they had a mind of their own. My family could no longer protect me from the truth. The outside world had already labeled me, and the worst part was that I started believing it. A new sense of self-loathing haunted me like a dark shadow, reminding me of my frailties, of my dysfunction that no one could name and, worse, no one could cure.

The only way to silence this self-doubt was to hit something, anything. It was the perfect Band-Aid over an infected wound. With every strike, a part of my innocence peeled away. Clearly, sooner or later I had to stop my violent outbreaks before I lost myself, but how?

Finally, to prevent any future episodes, my Pop sat me down and had a talk with me...mano-a-mano. Hell, someone had to. "You can't just act out like this, son. I promise we're gonna find out what's wrong," he said sternly. "But we can't afford to fix the walls and doors anymore."

Unfortunately, Pop's plea had little effect, as my blowups continued and, although hesitant, Pop resorted to an old-fashioned strategy. More often than not, his work belt lashed across my backside, and after Pop's whippings, I'd run into my room and curl up in my bed.

As I recalled Pop's words, I'd sometimes beat on my pillow—a more advantageous, softer choice. "I'm so sorry, son, but you gotta control that temper of yours," he would say, before yanking off his belt.

Each strike of leather stirred my silent fury even more. *It's not my fault*, I silently cried out.

On one particular evening, as I wept in my bunk, my brother slammed his book shut and leaned over his upper bunk. Pointing at me, he giggled. "You got in trouble. You got in trouble..." Over and over he taunted me.

Desperately, I shoved two pillows to the sides of my head and covered my ears. With my eyes shut, I imagined my fist pulverizing his face, but I knew what the repercussions would be if I attempted such a vengeful act. There would be no TV for a week, and my action figures would be taken away. I'd be belted once again. It just wasn't worth it.

As I tried to suppress my temper, Momma would walk on eggshells when dealing with me. She offered more extreme coddling than before—there were more forced smiles and increased protection from the phones and doorbells. She gave me tighter hugs, assuring me she loved me as I painstakingly tried to utter a word.

More than once, I overheard Momma's whispered plea to the family, "Let's not make him mad today, okay?" But I didn't have any animosity towards Momma's whispers behind my back and her desperate attempt to soothe my hostility. She tried to deal with me the only way she could, saturating me with love like a good Sicilian mother. And at the very least, her persistent enabling might have succeeded in saving her walls from further destruction. Or it might have been a way of keeping me from a dismal date with Pop's belt. Perhaps she was trying to save me from myself.

Ironically, I had begun to change, not only physically, but also psychologically into The Hulk—well, at least the more human side of him. Like Dr. Bruce Banner—The Hulk's alter ego—I had to control my rage so I wouldn't turn into some monstrosity who inflicted terror and fear upon his loved ones. Bruce Banner's infamous line from the television show constantly rang in my head: "Don't make me angry; you wouldn't like me when I'm angry!" This was a tall order for a young stutterer trying to cope.

To protect my family from my looming eruptions, I lived in isolation. Like a deaf-mute, I shut off vocally. After all, if I didn't talk, I wouldn't lose my temper. If I wanted something, I'd point. If I meant no, I'd shake my head.

Within my voluntary solitude, I kept my mind active by conjuring up tangible fantasies. With the help of my action figures, I reenacted scenarios not of galactic heroism, but of real life incidents. Sometimes, I'd ram The Hulk into Vader. The Hulk represented me. Darth Vader was Pop. Like a skipping record, the scenario of me giving Pop a whipping kept replaying in my mind. I saw Pop's belt swatting down on him, my hand firmly holding the end of the belt. Perhaps a part of my indignation stemmed from my hidden resentment toward my parents for not explaining what was wrong with me, leaving me in the dark until it was too late.

But there was one individual in the house who made sense of it all, who made me feel like a normal boy. Momma Nettie had looked past my bloody knuckles and my crimson, raged face because she identified with my turmoil. Fighting lonesome battles was in her DNA. She didn't buy into the coddling of a boy who fought against an undefined dysfunction. Instead, she saw a boy who longed to be heard and understood. Momma Nettie knew all too well about being misunderstood.

Some nights, after the dishes were done and Pop and Momma slipped under their covers, Momma Nettie would tell me to come into her room. "You're sleeping with me tonight." Lacing her cigarette-stained fingers through mine as we lay on her bed, Nettie had her other hand wrapped around a glass of scotch and 7-Up. She'd click on *Quincy* and *Columbo*, and we'd escape from our hardships, losing ourselves in characters that were just as underestimated as we were.

Before she made me say my nightly prayers, Nettie kissed my forehead and reassured me, "You're my baby. My little bust 'em up. No matter what, you're going to get through whatever you got. Your problems become God's blessings. Remember that."

As her words of hope rocked me to sleep, I'd dream of being older and speaking in front of a large crowd. Sporting a three-piece suit and standing in front of a podium, I spoke effortlessly, while the words flowed out of my mouth in perfect tempo. The eyes of a massive audience were locked onto me. I had something pressing, almost monumental to say. I didn't remember the words, but I did recall the feeling I possessed as I spoke, each word an example of grace and elegance. I had a purpose. I had a place in the world. My words were transforming everyone within hearing distance.

When I was awake and living my real life, Momma's worries intensified as my stammering worsened. Attempting to express myself once again and break free from the chains of silence, my words lodged further in my throat, and a frantic crackling sound followed. Instead of punching walls and doors, I found a new way of dealing with my stress. My foot would kick the nearest thing next to it—a chair, a wall, or a low cabinet in the kitchen lay victim to my frustration.

The coddling wasn't working. Neither were the spankings or the reassurance from Momma Nettie that everything was going to turn out for the best. Something had to be done.

At first, I didn't know what Momma meant when she told me we had a doctor's appointment. *Is it the dentist? Is it a check-up with our pediatrician?* My young mind played Twenty Questions as I watched Momma laying out my church clothes on the bed.

I buttoned up my blue dress shirt, zipped up the khaki pants, and slipped on my freshly polished shoes. Minutes later in the bathroom, Momma slicked my hair back and smiled, "You look so handsome, son."

I studied myself in the mirror. I looked as if I was dressed for Christmas mass. I asked, "Wh-Wh-Where are we g-g-g..."

Setting the comb down, Momma cut me off, "We're going to see somebody who may know how to help you." Perhaps her eagerness in where we were going made her interrupt me, or perhaps she couldn't listen to one more stammer come out of my mouth. Whatever the reason, she beamed with excitement, and that calmed my curiosity.

4 Buffers

"Oh, you should never, never doubt what nobody is sure about."
—*Willy Wonka*

The dull gray colored walls and the flickering fluorescent bulbs unnerved me as we entered the clinic. Momma led me to a wooden door that had some complex wording on it. Because of my limited reading ability, I didn't know the meaning of the words, but later I would find out what those words represented, for they symbolized my first steps along a lengthy, strenuous journey to find my voice. We had arrived at "The Jefferson Speech and Language Center."

Because of the public's growing awareness of dyslexia, dysgraphia, dyscalculia, and other learning disorders in the late '60s, The Jefferson Speech and Language Center (JSLC)—named after the parish in which it was located—was founded in 1972 to help assist with the reading deficiencies plaguing New Orleans schools. Due to the limited recognition of stuttering in the late '70s, my parents thought JSLC could well be the best local center to help us find answers. After Momma's many calls and inquiries, JSLC finally advised us to come in for a consultation.

At the time, few of the pathologists on staff dealt extensively with stuttering, but after giving me a series of tests, JSLC could refer us to the most suitable pathologist in the area. Little did I know that Momma and Pop had already been looking at a plethora of centers across the country, and had set some money aside for my rehabilitation.

For months, brochures and packets filtered into our house from the various speech institutes. The Hollins Communication Research Institute (HCRI) was number one on my parents' shortlist of places in the nation that offered extensive therapy. Founded in the early '70s as the leading institute in stuttering, HRCI offered an array of cutting-edge techniques for moderate to severe stutterers.

But my parents' plans for me to attend this illustrious institute had hit some snags. For one, the cost of such a school exceeded my family's budget. Pop had just opened his mechanic business, and my parents' future economic stability remained in question. Plus, HRCI was located in Virginia. Depending on the severity of my stuttering, Momma and I would have to relocate to Roanoke for one to three months, living out of a hotel room. This meant that Momma would be missing out on work, and I would have to skip kindergarten, which meant I'd be a year behind.

In addition, the price of a hotel stay would surely put a hole in my family's budget. We were left with limited options—that is, until JSLC came into our lives.

Sitting across a desk from a JSLC doctor, I held my breath, not knowing what to expect. Momma sat in the corner, observing me during the initial meeting. The calm, reserved doctor asked me some procedural questions. After my responses, she scribbled on her notepad:

"Do you love your parents?"

"Y-Y-Yes."

"Are you happy?"

"N-N-No"

"Why?"

"I t-t-talk f-f-f…"

"Funny?"

I nodded. I was afraid that if I didn't answer correctly, I'd be punished. I picked at my fingernails as I stared at the shut door. How I wanted to leave! I longed to go home and watch Bob Barker with Momma Nettie. But there was no escape, no timeout as my consultation continued.

Audible tests followed, one involving repeating words after the doctor stated them. I found following the rhythm of someone who spoke fluently was a daunting experience. The doctor could say the word, but I knew that, ultimately, I couldn't. This test sent me spiraling into a frantic state, which forced me to use my coping weapon of choice, my "buffers."

To compensate for my stuttering, I had recently created a desperate remedy by placing "um" and "ah" in between letters when I felt the tension billowing up in my throat. The buffers gave me a moment to gather my thoughts and appear slightly normal. When I overheard adults, I witnessed them using "ah" and "um" when speaking, as if they were subconsciously taking time for their mouths to catch up with their thoughts. It seemed as if everyone used buffers, and practicing such a contrivance gave me a feeling of normalcy.

But my buffers were premeditated, a feeble tool to conceal my dysfunction so I could come across as a "normal" speaker. It would be one of the many ineffective methods I created to cope with my stuttering.

"Fries," said the doctor.

I repeated, "F-F-F-um, um, um, F-F-F, um, um, ries."

"Orange"

"O-o-o-o-ah-um-ah-o-o-o-range."

During the testing, my compulsive side forced me to go back and repeat the word to make sure I got it right, and to prove to the doctor and to Momma that I could get it right. But every time I returned to a troubled letter, it would stick harder, longer. The tests seemed impossible. Here and there, I heard some encouraging words from Momma, like, "That's my big boy."

I knew she had to say such supportive words, but I didn't believe her. Surely she noticed the sweat rings under my arms, and my fidgety hands fumbling about, as the nervous swaying of my body rocked me back and forth like a pendulum. I couldn't see her, but I felt Momma's anxieties pressing in on me. Hearing her little boy repeat words as he struggled and stumbled must have been an excruciating experience for her.

After the series of repetitions, the examiner produced pictures of simple objects. She asked me to identify them orally. Hearing a word and repeating it was one thing, but for me to see a picture and have to articulate it without someone's vocal example was nearly impossible.

As my stuttering swelled during this rigorous exercise, something significant came to light. Besides the progression of my stuttering, I also omitted "th" and "d" when they appeared in the middle of a word.

For instance, instead of saying "ladder" when I saw it on a picture card, I would say "l-l-l-um-laer," or instead of "birthday cake," I'd sputter out, "b-b-bir-um-biray c-c-ah-cake." Somehow, my nerves and my articulation heightened more when I had to conjure up the word. I had hit a huge, telling, and very troublesome spot.

As we finished up the grueling two-hour tests, I slumped in the chair, exhausted. After inviting Momma to stay in the office, the examiner guided me out the door and asked me to sit in the waiting room. While my feet dangled from the chair, I stared at the closed door to the office, overhearing the mumbled voices of Momma and the doctor seeping from under the door.

Even though I couldn't understand their words, clearly I was the topic of conversation. Pressing my hands over my ears, I tried to silence their mumbled words. *You failed*, I told myself. But what I didn't realize was that I had, at last, taken my first real step toward recovery.

Our drive from the Center seemed less encouraging than our drive out there that morning. What seemed like an answer to our problem had become a more complicated situation, not only for me, but for Momma as well. In the car, Momma didn't make a sound as we made our way home. This was out of character for such a normally opinionated and outspoken woman. Instead, Momma kept looking out the driver's window, hiding her puffy eyes and sniffling nose.

To break the silence, I did the only thing I could do to comfort her. I grabbed Momma's clammy hand and squeezed hard. She turned and graced me with the best smile she could summon, "Everything's fine, baby. You're going to be fine."

Even at four and a half years old, I knew a lie when I heard one.

5 I'm a Stutterer

"Everybody is a stranger, but that's the danger in going my own way."
—John Mayer

That night, following our visit to the Center, the house smelled like a four-star restaurant. Momma whipped up an exceptional meal that exceeded our budget. Like any ethnic household that revered cooking and eating as a therapeutic distraction, our house was of no exception. Momma's impromptu feast released some of the emotional strain we experienced with the doctor that morning. The scent of garlic from the meat and potatoes permeated throughout the entire house.

Five thick steaks and a huge pot of cheese-mashed potatoes were on the menu, and everyone welcomed the scrumptious surprise. Well, everyone, except for Pop, who usually worked into the late hours of the night at his mechanic shop.

As the rest of my family sat around the table cutting into their steaks with joyous commitment, smiles exuded from around the table. I, on the other hand, sat there, skeptical. Unable to enjoy my festive dinner, I studied Momma's face across from me. Her forced smile and spur-of-the-moment meal choice told me that she was concealing something. I may have been young, but my sensitivity was as seasoned as the steak I bit into.

As I tossed and turned in bed, a silent caution thumped in my head, and I wondered what Momma hadn't shared with me after her meeting with the doctor. Would I ever be privy to the cause of my dysfunction? Or more importantly, would I ever know the name of my dysfunction?

Later that night, Pop came home from work. The rustling of his keys and his deep cadence woke me from my semi-slumber. Staring up at the ceiling, I tried to hear my parents' garbled conversation, so I crept out of my room to hear more clearly. Yes, it was a grave sin to eavesdrop on adults and their conversations, but I had become desperate. Hiding in the shadows of the hallway, I overheard Momma and Pop's clandestine discussion about the doctor's assessment. Complex terminologies were thrown around like Frisbees; phrases that boggled my mind, "mumbled diction when reciting words...face contortions...Scotty is outgoing...his dysfunction must be taken care of...."

The jargon was cluttered and foreign, as if my parents spoke Aramaic. Then I heard the words that would become the subtitle to my existence, the words that would categorize me for the rest of my life. "The doctor determined that Scott is a severe stutterer."

Stutterer. I am a severe stutterer. A new complex meaning to my being had been forged. It sounded like extra-terrestrial words, like something out of *Star Wars*. I slumped over in the hallway, staring into the darkness of my future, trying to piece everything together, trying to make sense of it all. I couldn't comprehend any of it, except for that one word that ricocheted in my head — stutterer. The freak had a title now. Never did I want to hit a wall so badly.

In that dank hallway, I had been baptized into the ranks of many throughout history who tussled and agonized with the idea of being labeled a stutterer. The confusion that followed me throughout my life only mirrored the tormented souls who preceded me. In Greek times, stuttering was as enigmatic and dreaded as leprosy. Many believed stuttering was linked to demonic possessions. Centuries later, scholars testify that Moses placed hot coals on his tongue to control his stuttering, so he could carry out the word of God with fluency. The Great Emperor Claudius was ostracized by the public and ultimately from his throne due to his severer stuttering. In the eighteenth and nineteenth centuries, doctors resorted to slicing the tongue, or removing the uvula and tonsils as a way of curtailing the stuttering. But time proved these methods to be barbaric, as well as masochistic. Thus, the age of therapy came into play during the twentieth century. Pathologists took the reins and brought a more rational and logical approach to the dysfunction. I thank God I was never born prior to 1901.

Weeks after my consultation, we visited various speech pathologists based on JSLC's referrals. During that time, Momma and Pop explained my deficiency to me with careful, simple words. For the most part, they reassured me that they would do everything in their power to find a cure. But having the right intentions didn't guarantee the right answers.

Searching for a compatible pathologist was like searching for a soul mate. Do we speak the same language? Is there chemistry? Do they understand my needs? After our first sessions with various doctors, my stuttering usually increased, which confused us even more. How could meeting with pathologists have a counteractive result? Most of the time, after she realized a doctor wasn't helping, Momma would ask me, "I don't think he's working out, do you?" I'd shake my head. Thus, we'd move on to the next pathologist on our list.

I remember one particular visit with a pathologist. In the office mirror, I stared at my lips, making dramatic formations with my mouth as I punched each letter of the alphabet. Resembling a fish gasping for his last breath, I puckered my lips, stammering and stumbling on most of the consonants.

With his reflection staring back at me, the pathologist stood behind me, giving a slight nod as if I was progressing in my exercise. But, in my opinion, I wasn't getting any better. I knew it. Momma knew it. Over and over we would go over this mundane drill. I loathed myself when I stuttered, but looking at my reflection while stuttering exasperated me even more.

To my disappointment, every pathologist we visited consistently instilled this regiment. I wondered if they all took orders from the same itinerary. Was there a meeting amongst the pathologists, where a lead doctor stood behind a long table and exclaimed, "You know, we should have patients make those weird faces in the mirror. That'll help, right?"

Another exercise involved my body going rigid, every muscle pulsating with tension. Complying with the doctor's orders, I'd tighten my whole body into a state of flexing, squeezing until my limbs went numb. When the pathologist counted to ten, I'd release, allowing my muscles into a state of relaxation. Then I'd do it again, building the tension, and then releasing. For ten minutes this activity continued as the pathologist hummed, "Yeeeees, veeeery goooood."

His voice vibrated from a lower register, resembling the tone of a New Age guru. Sensing my annoyance, the doctor explained that this exercise would help me relax more when I spoke, but all I got in return was an achy stomach and the sudden need to release my bladder.

During those early years, pathologists came in and out of my life like busboys, yet none had a lasting effect on me. I didn't blame them for their lack of help, or for the monotonous exercises that led to a stalemate. Even today, their faces and features rush past my thoughts; I can still see their eager expressions, and their urge to help a kid in need. But they didn't know the complicated nature of my stammering. Perhaps my problem didn't stem from the physical aspects of how I spoke, like a disconnection between my mouth and brain, or the misplacement of my tongue. Perhaps a deeper, more psychological reason triggered my stuttering—an unforeseen, visceral reaction to something that lingered in the dark.

As the search for the quintessential therapist seemed futile, the time had come to start my formal schooling. Starting kindergarten would have made any stutterer cringe—strange kids, a new social setting, the umbilical cord of home severed. But to my surprise—and my parents' as well—I eased into my first formal year of education, even though my self-doubt lingered in the back of my head. Having a pathologist privy to my stuttering was one thing, but having unforgiving, five and six-year-old kids witness my embarrassing dilemma was something entirely different. So I made it my mission to keep my hidden foe a secret as I interacted with my classmates. To do this, I put on a big show, a persona that included a broad smile, giddy laughter, and an unceasing participation in physical activities. I didn't know it at the time, but I was starting to perform, creating a "me" to disguise my silent shame.

In class, my dysfunction was kept at a minimum during our formal drills. For instance, when we recited the ABC's in concert, my stuttering never occurred. When hearing others speak the word while I said it with them, I was never held accountable, never pointed out. The pressure was off my shoulders, and I took great delight in this revelation.

On the schoolyard, I pushed my body to run faster and dodge balls with more dexterity than my peers. Unconsciously, I knew if I was judged by my athletic attributes instead of my speaking abilities, then my peers would accept me. Thus, my strategies proved foolproof, as my classmates consistently chose me for their dodge ball games or hide-and-seek.

Interacting with other students had its ups and downs. I stammered here and there, yet I kept my responses to one or two words. Mostly I listened, never involving myself in lengthy conversations.

Soon school friends turned into neighborhood friends. Playing war and climbing trees became our weekend activities. I never knocked on doors or asked if someone could come out and play for fear of exposing my shameful flaw. Instead, I waited for the right opportunity to present itself. Every Saturday morning as I gulped down my two bowls of cereal, I peered through the curtains and skimmed the neighborhood, hoping to find kids who were playing outside. If they were running about the street, I darted out the front door and jumped into their games. A wave or a smile was all I had to give them, nothing audible or vocally challenging. They knew me from class. They knew me as the smiley kid in the red brick house who hardly said a word but participated in anything and everything.

Seeing their introverted son transform into a social butterfly whose temper had simmered, my parents ceased their search for the right pathologist, and Momma stopped her coddling. Perhaps I would outgrow my speech impediment after all. Perhaps the stammering was just part of my stumbling pursuit to find my voice. Perhaps the Center we visited months ago had it all wrong.

6 The Schemes

"Truly it is an evil to be full of faults; but it is a still greater evil to be full of them and to be unwilling to recognize them, since that is to add the further fault of a voluntary illusion."
— Blaise Pascal

After a summer filled with swimming at the local YMCA and playing street soccer with the neighborhood kids, I returned to school. For the first time since answering the phone a year and a half prior, I felt like a normal and accepted kid during those summer days of carefree. But the first-grade called, and with it, a dose of reality.

First grade's strict protocols sent me for a loop. Instead of casually sitting on the floor like we did in kindergarten, my class was ordered to sit alphabetically in desks according to our last names. We were assigned bulky, wordy books that intimidated me more than anything else. The intensity of schooling went from zero to sixty in the blink of an eye, and I wasn't prepared for the formality of it all.

When it came to private schools in the greater New Orleans area, St. Benilde was as parochial as any institution. While attending Kindergarten, I heard of Benilde's strict discipline in grades one through eight, yet never experienced it up close until my brother—already four grades ahead of me—repeatedly dashed home, crying and carrying a report that documented his "excessive need to interrupt class." I saw firsthand how a ruler could tattoo a nine-year-old boy's hand—long red lines on the knuckles that resembled stripes on a peppermint stick. If the nuns and priests of St. Benilde unleashed their wrath on my brother for his interruptions, surely they would rain fire and brimstone upon me for speaking funny in class, or so I thought. Being Catholic had some side effects which included guilt—guilt even when the innocent was innocent.

Relief came when I found out a laywoman was teaching my first grade class. Having someone outside the cloth calmed my nerves, especially when that aforementioned laywoman was Ms. Marquez. Marquez's petite and gentle voice mirrored her patient and kind personality. She didn't wield a ruler, or intimidate to control her class. Her patience always prevailed, and I thought her tolerance would prove beneficial for me when it came to hiding my dysfunction.

It was our second or third week of class, and Ms. Marquez stood in front of the chalkboard, and said, "I hope you all read the pages that were assigned to you yesterday." Heads nodded around the class. "Good, 'cause now we are going to read those pages out loud."

Staring at Marquez, I couldn't help but feel contempt for her. She didn't know it, but she gave an order that could possibly crush my reputation, and lead me to the principal's office. My heart skipped a beat. My sights fixed on the unopened book that sat on my desk. I couldn't crack it open. I dared not look at the words. Reading with harmonious voices was one thing, but reading alone was something entirely different.

Pointing at my row, Ms. Marquez said, "We will go alphabetically and start with this row." I sat fourth in the row.

The first student started his slow, careful approach to the reading. Giggles chimed in around the class. If they were laughing at his slight hesitation, I couldn't bear to think of what type of response awaited me as I stammered my way through the assignment. Out of the corner of my eye, I saw the door, my way out. Without even thinking, my hand shot up.

Ms. Marquez recognized me, "What is it, Scott?"

Jittering like a cranked up toy, I tried to formulate the word that was in my thoughts. *Bathroom.* Ever since I could remember, there were certain letters that made me cringe, troubling letters that appeared at the beginning or in the middle of a word; letters that I called "bad no-no's." These paralyzing letters were impossible to pronounce without stammering. Among the distressing letters on my list, which included many consonants, "B" was a big bad no-no.

In what seemed like forever, I fixed on that "B" as I nervously held up my hand. I was certain that once I overcame the "B," then I could move on to the next letters of the word more easily. But that friggin' "B" cornered me from my freedom.

All eyes locked on me. "You can lower your hand, Scott, and tell me what you want," said Ms. Marquez.

A raspberry fluttered between my lips. I pushed again. "Um...um...ah." The buffers weren't helping. Another raspberry followed. *B...say it...B!* Suddenly, I came up with another word; a synonym that not only caught me off guard, but also distracted me from the troubled word.

"P-P-Potty!" I exclaimed. Instinctually, the word spewed forth. I had psyched myself out, and in the process, tricked my voice and head into a word I didn't dwell upon. Yet out it came, clear and with no stammer. Sure "potty" was an infantile word used in Kindergarten, but at least I got my point across and freed myself from a more horrid disaster like reading out loud in class.

Ms. Marquez pointed to the door. Bolting out the door, a momentary relief came over me. I could breathe easily. But most importantly, I devised another way to skirt around my stuttering. By inventing synonyms for words that stumped me—especially words that started with bad no-no's—I could articulate without the contortion of my face or the long, embarrassing guttural sounds. Like buffers, substituting words—which I later called "replacers"—became a valuable coping mechanism for the rest of my stuttering life, and yet, the more I used replacers, the more it halted my progress.

Weaseling my way from reading aloud became a recurring event; a stressful game that forced me to devise other inventive ploys. I continued to raise my hand right before my turn came up.

Sometimes I'd use replacers like "Toilet," or "Wee-wee." The classmates would laugh at my unsophisticated words, but I didn't care. I had dodged a bullet.

On a few occasions, I wouldn't even use a word. I'd point to the door, and let Ms. Marquez deduce my meaning, which soon became our own version of charades. After Ms. Marquez gave me permission to go and relieve myself, I'd haul ass to the bathroom. In one of the three stalls, I waited five to ten minutes before returning to class, which proved enough time for my teacher to skip over me.

Another tactic entailed holding my stomach, and moaning in class. Marquez asked if I was okay. I responded with a shake of the head. "To the nurse's office you go," she commanded. My pseudo-medical scheme bought me at least a half an hour to let the reading commence without me. Drinking the nasty Pepto-Bismol in front of the nurse seemed like a small price to pay.

At times, I'd fake a cough, and wave my hand in the air. I pointed to my throat, implying I couldn't stop. Ordering me to the water fountain, Marquez reluctantly allowed me to leave class.

Sometimes the grace of timing and pure luck helped me escape humiliation. This grace came in the form of a ringing bell, declaring the end of class. Like a game show, I stared at the clock above the chalkboard, praying that God would make that bell clang before my turn to read aloud arrived. Intensely, I'd watch the little hand click its way to my liberation.

I tried everything under the sun to escape reading out loud, and all proved highly successful. The only scam I didn't perform was a disappearing act, but I was working on it. Nevertheless, I had hit upon infallible schemes. Maybe I could carry on these ruses for the rest of my academic career. But, little did I know, my newfound acting abilities weren't enough to bamboozle a savvy teacher like Ms. Marquez.

To make a more viable relationship between parents and teachers, St. Benilde scheduled monthly parent/teacher conferences. As my parents' first appointment with Ms. Marquez neared, I was more than certain my first-grade teacher would deliver a satisfactory report to Momma and Pop.

I couldn't have been farther from the truth.

During the conference—which I would discover years later— Ms. Marquez asked my parents if I suffered from any type of anxiety when it came to reading out loud. My parents explained how I had been diagnosed as a severe stutterer and that I, quite possibly, was making up excuses as a copout. Instead of being indignant to my behavior, Ms. Marquez offered my parents advice that would change my complicated world.

As I waited impatiently for my parents to come home from the meeting, I imagined them barging through the door in a song of praise for their son who had gone above and beyond their expectations. Rather, returning home, my parents expressed their grave disappointment at my surreptitious schemes.

"It's the same as lying, son," my Pop said.

Knowing that my furtive actions caused my parents' disappointment, I couldn't look at them as my eyes scanned the floor. They were right, but what other choice did I have? There was no way I could face the class with an impediment that would surely earn me ridicule. My heart couldn't take such rejection. I had worked so hard on my reputation as an athletic, joyous boy who seemed perfect in every way. In my limited scope, it was better to lie.

As my mind raced a mile a minute, Momma gently offered another consolation, "Your teacher knows about your stuttering, and she understands. And so do we. She gave us the number of someone who may be able to help us. She's across the river, but we can meet with her and see what she has to offer."

"Wh-Wh-What's her n-n-n-name," I struggled to ask.

Reaching into her purse, Momma took out a folded piece of paper. She unwrinkled it, and read from it. "Dr. Hambuga."

7 The Savior in the Trailer

"If I cannot fly, let me sing."
—Stephen Sondheim

If we knew how vital she would be in my recovery, we would have driven to Istanbul to get to her. But how could we have known? Still, there was an air of skepticism on our forty-minute drive to see Dr. Hambuga. We had been through it before; the barrage of questions thrown at me, the extensive exercises, the excuses we had to tell the pathologist about why we couldn't participate in further appointments, and the frustration that ensued.

According to Ms. Marquez, Dr. Hambuga was one of those few pathologists in the area who focused primarily on stuttering, even though her name never appeared on JSLC's shortlist. Dr. Hambuga's office was a large air-conditioned trailer that stood on concrete blocks. An odd choice, but I was struck by her decor. Like her approach to speech impediments, Dr. Hambuga's surroundings exuded warmth. Festive pastel couches and chairs furnished the trailer, and cartooned illustrations of mouth and tongue placements graced her wooden-paneled walls. Posters of happy children running and leaping about were pinned to the doors. Under the jubilant posters were the words, "By My Smile I Look Normal To You, So Why Would You Judge Me Any Other Way?"

Radiating charisma, Dr. Hambuga welcomed me as I made my way into her office. The scent of the trailer reminded me of my family's pop-up camper. *It smells like vacation*, I thought. The floorboards creaked with each step she took. Shaking her hand, my fingers looked like twigs compared to her mitts. Her laid back attire of a Hawaiian shirt, khaki pants, and flip-flops lightened my apprehension.

Leading me into her office, Dr. Hambuga asked Momma to come back in an hour. "He's in good hands." Not having Momma there felt like I was about to tread water without my floaties. But once she left, the flushness to my face dissipated when Hambuga peered down at me and said in a congenial voice, "Well, it's just you and me, kiddo. How 'bout we have some fun?"

She clapped her hands and gave a jovial chuckle as if we were about to delve into some mischief. I was game.

Guiding me to a table filled with picture cards, an array of books, and a jar full of lollipops, Hambuga pointed to an open book. Seven lines of a poem stared back at me. "I'd love to hear this poem. Could you read it for me?" she asked.

An unwelcome dread hit my gut—that damn reading out loud again. I wanted to get the words right. I wanted to make a grand first impression. The desperation on my face must have been evident, because Hambuga flashed me a sympathetic smile. "You're fine. It's going to be fine," she said, resting her hand on my back and melting my chill-ridden nerves. "Just take a deep breath, and let go. It's okay. You're safe here."

You're safe here. Her soothing words instantaneously dissolved most of the tension from my small frame. I began the poem. The stammering slapped from the back of my mouth. As I struggled through the poem, my habitual self-awareness came into play once again, and I focused less on what I was reading and more on how I sounded and appeared.

When someone witnessed my stuttering, they probably assumed I had palsy. It couldn't have been comfortable to watch my head pop to and fro, as my eyes rolled back, eyelids shuttering, throat gargling, face bending and contorting, and my body clenching. Yet, to my surprise, when my involuntary symptoms persisted in front of Dr. Hambuga, all she did was rub my upper back, and impart words of encouragement, "Nice, Scott. You're doing well. Work through it...you got it."

Her words weren't patronizing in the least. At six years old, I could detect insincerity when I heard it. Hambuga meant her words. She understood me, and that was all I asked from anyone. My unorthodox sounds and unsettling head movements must have been a normal occurrence for Hambuga. Other kids with similar deficiencies probably marched in and out of her trailer door on a consistent basis. The only evidence of their existence lay in their crayoned pictures that hung above the table. I visualized those nameless kids in my head, desperately wanting to meet them, to connect with them, to color with them, and to compare my unique impairment with theirs.

Once I finished the poem, a proud smile emanated from Hambuga's pudgy face. "You did it, kiddo! You got through the poem. Good job!"

At first, I didn't know why Hambuga congratulated me for my flawed effort, but her sincere thrill was contagious. After a while, it sunk in that she was right. I had done something monumental. I read out loud for the first time in the presence of someone else, and I had survived it. I glanced over at the poster of the kids smiling. I felt like one of them, and I quietly repeated the poster's rhetorical question, *so why would you judge me any other way?*

For our next exercise, Hambuga positioned five reading cards in front of me. Each card had a vowel on it. "This may seem trivial, but I want you to sing the letters on these cards. I bet you have a great voice, don't you?"

I nodded.

"I could tell," she remarked with a wink.

Taking in a deep breath and conjuring up my best singing voice, I opened my mouth and glided through the vowels, "AAAAAAAA-EEEEEEEEE-IIIIIIIII-OOOOOOOO-UUUUUUU."

Each word skated past my tongue. My heart fluttered. An energetic jolt shot through my bones. I had just recited five letters without stuttering, including "E," which was one of my bad no-

no's. I stared at Dr. Hambuga in awe. A few minutes ago, she was a complete stranger. Now she was a magician, a goddess, and a savior.

"Nicely done!" she declared. "Those are your bridges. Vowels are the bridges between consonants. Think of that when we read aloud the next time we see each other. Now, let's go through the vowels again, yes?"

Because of my exhilaration after our first session, further appointments followed with the pathologist in the trailer. Hambuga and I met once a week, and I looked forward to each meeting because I was always discovering and pushing. Sometimes I'd have homework assignments. Other times, Hambuga requested Momma's participation in my take-home exercises.

While working through the exercises at the dinner table, Momma and I bonded in a profound way. Her patience shined and my appreciation for her intensified. Finally, we were making progress, and we were accomplishing something together. In unison, we sang the words and the names of pictures printed on flash cards—our voices sounding like an *a cappella* opera. During those melodious feats, I felt invincible, like I could say anything. I crushed the bad no-no's with one swoop of my vibrato.

It wasn't long until I carried my lyrical exercise into my normal day communication. Whenever I sang full sentences to convey an emotion or a need, my family patiently listened; a smile sprang from them, as a more cheerful stare followed. They welcomed any type of game plan that would lend to my improvement. Yet a question lingered behind their joyous responses: What would happen in the real world when I couldn't sing my words?

There were physiological reasons why I didn't stutter when going into a song. Using my melodic voice, the right side of my brain instantly took over. The right side controls any creative output—acting, painting, and dancing—where the left side is used more for conversing or analytical thinking. Researchers believe when stutterers shift to the right side of the brain, more fluency is produced.

Support from the diaphragm is also another relevant reason for lyrical fluency. Because my stuttering transpired from a constriction in the throat and mouth, singing relocated the tension from my oral region to my diaphragm—a more stable and grounded region for diction and projection. Also, when singing, air passes through the vocal cords with more ease, as compared to stuttering where the air is restricted by tension. The singing thus expands the vocal cords, allowing fluency to be permitted.

The right side of the brain, the diaphragm, and airflow—my three best allies for life, and all stimulated by singing. My limited comprehension couldn't understand these anatomical concepts at the time, but I welcomed the results, and so did my family for the time being.

Nearing the second month with my miracle worker, Momma and Hambuga scheduled a conference about my progress. While they quietly discussed my case, I sat in the corner of the trailer and went over assigned speech exercises. They didn't know it, but I passively listened in. By this time I had become a professional in overhearing adult chitchat, as I read lips and listened for key words. Guilt in doing so went out the window a while ago.

During their meeting, Hambuga expressed her assurance in my progression to my mother. Even though Momma agreed and felt more optimistic about my full recovery, she asked when I would be able to wean off the singing, and use a normal voice.

"In due time," Hambuga said. "He'll ease into it. But for now, let him enjoy it." Hambuga was right. I was enjoying my tuneful speech, and because of it, the rage diminished. My parents finally had their kid back.

A few minutes later, Hambuga went a step further with the conversation. She delved deeper into the psychological reasons behind my stuttering, which included my tendency to get in my own way when speaking, and how my acute self-awareness hindered my confidence. Her words hung like wet clothes, slapping around in my head. All this psychobabble weighed heavily on me. I still felt like a problem child, and I didn't want to be anyone's problem.

In her pensive tone, Momma asked Hambuga to expound more on her theory.

"Scott is one of those cases where he knows he will stutter. When he speaks or reads out loud, he instantly believes he will stutter before he opens his mouth."

What pinched me the most from Hambuga's assessment was that I knew she was right. I had created my own dilemmas, and the heartache that my family endured was caused by my sabotaging ways. My bad no-no's were a prime example of how I incapacitated myself before I even opened my mouth. I believed in my failure before I had time to override the failure.

"We have a lot of work to do," Hambuga continued, "But once Scott gets a handle on his stuttering, and more comfortable with his voice...and I know he will...who knows how much will come out of that boy."

Like she did many times before, Hambuga's assurance nourished my troubled mind. A ray of hope shone in the corner of the trailer, where most of my dreams and aspirations were buried deep under the methodical exercises, which lay before me. I had choices. I had a way out, but was I willing to see them through?

The doctor and Momma discussed other things, but I paid no mind after that. I had more pressing matters to attend to, like my chance for articulation. Softly, I sung to myself, "AAAAAAAA-EEEEEEEEE-IIIIIIIIII-OOOOOOOO-UUUUUUU."

On our way home from Hambuga's office, Momma stopped at Burger King and ordered me a hamburger. It was my reward for what she called, "a challenging few weeks." We sat in a large orange booth and nibbled on French fries. I unwrapped my cheeseburger and glared at it for some time. Quietly, I mouthed the word, "H-A-M-B-U-R-G-E-R."

The word had a new meaning. It sounded like the name of a woman who gave me my first taste of confidence through all the chaos. I bit into the sandwich, and savored the juicy patty. A "hambuga" never tasted so good.

8 A Side Order of Stupidity

"There's a fine line between courage and foolishness. Too bad it's not a fence."
—Anonymous

Even years later, I can't pinpoint the genesis for my foolish idea to read out loud. There was a throng of reasons behind my plan. For one, Hambuga's optimism boosted my enthusiasm into high gear. And the movies I habitually watched, where good guys always won, added to my firm resolution that life did have happy endings. Whatever the reason, I was ready to make that next step to prove my voice. But for a six year old in 1979, my flights of fantasy spun out of control, and overrode the reality that would once again snare me in its claws.

Nestled under my covers at night, I envisioned my reading in front of the class, with no fears attached, and no hesitation to my demeanor. Once I punched out my last word with articulation, the kids would cheer for me, carry me on their shoulders, and declare me as one of them. Every minute of the day I prayed that my nighttime dreams would come into fruition.

But in the classroom, I never had the opportunity to put my aspirations into action. After the first parent-teacher conference, Ms. Marquez unfailingly skipped over me when the reading out loud commenced. I assumed Momma had a discussion with my teacher, or perhaps Marquez and Hambuga spoke of my situation over coffee and beignets. Whatever the reason, I was grateful for my teacher's empathetic tendencies as she passed over me, while randomly choosing readers instead of going row by row. Yet, the more I heard other kids practicing and developing their reading skills, the more I became antsy, and longed to read like them in a normal and advanced fashion.

Walking the three blocks from my house to St. Benilde on a Friday morning, I set the plan in motion. My determination was firm as my shoes clomped up the steps to the school. *I am going to read out loud today.*

Approaching Ms. Marquez before class began, I asked her, "C-C-Could I r-r-read t-t-t-today?"

Her eyes widened, "Are you sure you're ready to do that?"

I nodded my head. By her narrow eyes and furrowed brow, I assumed she was wondering where all my courage and certitude derived from. Hell, I was asking myself the same question. Was it stubbornness or just plain stupidity that drove me to ask for such a request?

What Marquez didn't know—and what I wouldn't realize till years later—was that stubbornness ran rampant in my household; a family heirloom that I inherited from each member of my family, especially from Pop.

Almost every day, Momma's huffish comment, "That damn father of yours is a stubborn bastard, I swear," became a recurring opinion that echoed throughout the house. What I didn't know at the time were the specifics to Pop's stubbornness—a persistency that was deeply imbedded in his history.

In 1956, Pop had a few dollars to his name when he emigrated from Guatemala. As a teenager moving to New Orleans, Pop found harassment, heckles and hassles in the land of liberty, not only from whites, but also from blacks as well. Yet Pop was resilient. One day he would show those who beat him down that he wasn't just another "spic" off the boat. He would make a name for himself, beyond his bronze skin and his thick accent. Pop worked under cars for twelve hours a day; learning a blue-collar trade that gave him a sense of ownership. At the age of thirty-two, he opened his own business on the outskirts of

Metairie. The kid known as "Wetback" had become his own man, and his own boss. Finally, he had put those naysayers in their place.

The odds were against Pop, yet he never listened. Some called him foolish for opening his own business. He had no college degree, he came from the projects, and English was his second language. It was stubbornness with a side order of stupidity that drove Pop. Any sane person would—and did—advise him to play it safe and get in with a big corporation, or work for someone higher up the food chain. But Pop was determined, and he was all in. Every cent he and Momma owned went into his American Dream.

My inherited obstinacy was what I carried in my gut as I faced my first grade teacher. I had to leap head first into the unknown, so I could alleviate the burden from my family, and the pain they endured because of my fumbling mouth. Feeling sorry for myself had come to an end.

Later that day, as some random student read aloud, I could feel my turn approaching. Clutching my hands together, I tried to squeeze away the shakiness and shivers from my fingers. Hours prior, during our lunch period, I went into one of the bathroom stalls and sang out my ABC's. I stretched out my mouth, making dramatic oral formations. Hambuga's exercises helped me prepare as much as I could; now all I had to do was set it in motion.

I looked around the classroom and studied the faces of the different students. Soon my reading capabilities would blow them away as they took in every word I read with acceptance and awe-filled reverence. Finally, I would be proud by what I could do and not by what I could hide.

Ms. Marquez locked eyes with me. A reluctant look waked over her face as she said, "You're next, Scott."

I gave a slight nod back. I opened my mouth. Taking a deep breath, I focused on the first word in the paragraph—"Before." That damn "B" crept up and started laughing at me. I couldn't gain my composure as I suddenly lost it. A raspberry fluttered from between my lips as I pushed the word from out of my mouth. My head tilted back and forth in a violent manner. Spit spewed from my mouth, trying to get that damn "B" out. I couldn't use a replacer. Everyone was glaring at the same word I was having trouble pronouncing.

My instincts suddenly took over. A long, melodic "B" floated from my mouth. Then, the full word, "Beeeeefoooore."

But I couldn't stop there. I had already landed on my safety net. Thus, I started to sing the succeeding words, like I was reading off of sheet music. A full-out musical gushed from out of me. Suddenly, a laugh boomed from the back of the room, then another, and soon a cacophony of cheers followed. The singing had caused pandemonium in the classroom.

Beside herself, Ms. Marquez bolted from behind the desk and tried to simmer the noisy class. I wasn't sure if the frown plastered on her face was because of my eccentric approach to my reading, or the boisterous response from my classmates. Either way, I didn't want to find out the reason. All I wanted to do was make everything better.

My brain shifted from the right to the left. With the next sentence, I tried to say it in my own voice without singing. *You can't do this*, I convinced myself.

"P-P-P-P..." The popping sound that came out of my mouth was unparalleled. The violent shakes increased. My nerves were shot. In a matter of seconds, a silent lull encompassed the room. If the singing brought uncontrollable laughter, then my stuttering forced everyone to look on in horror. Abruptly, and predictably, more uproarious laughter filled the classroom. Even today, I can still feel those laughs shaking my bones, and wrenching the insides of a hollow six-year old body.

Before I knew it, I had already sprinted out of the room. As I raced down the hallway, I heard Ms. Marquez telling the class to settle down, but I didn't care anymore. Nothing could save me now. The damage was done. The giggles pulled on me, wrecking my stomach to full-blown nausea.

I headed to my safe haven, the bathroom stall. Gripping onto the sides of the stall, I wondered if I could ever return to class. How could I ever be the same? And what could possibly await me in the years to come with the students and faculty looking at me as a sideshow? Hambuga was foolish to think there was any sort of progression to my voice, and I was gullible enough to believe her. It would take more than stubbornness to win back the acceptance I once had from my peers. It would take an act of God.

9 Sketches

"I prefer drawing to talking. Drawing is faster, and leaves less room for lies."
— Le Corbusier

If being lonely were a major, I would've received my Ph.D. in loneliness when I entered the second grade. After embarrassing myself in Ms. Marquez's class, I despised having to show my face at school. The thought of reading out loud or even speaking to a classmate made me shiver with trepidation.

In response, I fed and nurtured a self-inflicted ostracism during my first and second grade sojourn. Silence fell upon my lips, and I reverted back to my gestures — a shake of the head meaning no, and a nod meaning yes. Shadowy corners of the playground became my refuge as I watched my classmates throw balls and cheer each other on. I used to be part of them — the tribal shouts, the high-fives, and the camaraderie. A part of me wanted to jump into the playground revelry, but even if I tried to join them, I'd still feel like an oddity in their eyes. Thus, my quietude became my only playmate.

Giving up all hope, I begged Momma to cancel all further appointments with Dr. Hambuga. What was the point? Even though I knew the pathologist had the best intentions, how could she save me from the humiliation of it all? Hambuga may have been a miracle worker, but she wasn't God. She couldn't prevent the snickers and the laughs coming my way. Screw her exercises, screw the optimism that came with her regiments, and screw me for thinking I could enunciate a bad no-no in front of a whole class. There was no way I could find the courage again.

To get my point across about not seeing Hambuga, I relapsed back to my slamming on walls and counter tops. Over the temper tantrums, Momma begged me to return to my sessions. Emphatically, I shook my head. I was shutting out everyone who ever wanted to help me. Once again, I felt like a problem child, and I didn't want to be anyone's problem. I'd cope and deal with the stuttering my way—using replacements, buffers, singing, and when necessary, silence.

Not knowing it at the time, impatience got the better part of me. I expected instant success once I pushed past my comfort zone. But to have the chutzpah to open my mouth in front of a class was a feat in itself. My immature mind didn't grasp the triumph in my bold action. Momma and Pop tried to put it into perspective, trying to convince me to be patient, and that Dr. Hambuga was helping in the long run. But I wasn't drinking the Kool-Aid. Youthful rashness blinded me, and I didn't see the reward in the journey. I just wanted a quick result.

No more did I dream of speaking eloquently in front of a large crowd, for it was just that, a silly dream. My mind fixated on other things—other facets I had more control over. Provoked by TV watching and comic books, I created a fantastical world of make-believe that seemed more tangible, saner, and more inviting than reality. And because of my unbridled inventions, I stumbled upon an art form that would transform my life for the better.

On weekends, as the kids in the neighborhood climbed trees and ran to the local convenient store to grab an ICEE, I glued myself to the TV. My pride and shame wouldn't allow me to bolt out the door and participate in neighborhood merriment. As a consolation, I sat on the couch with my brother and watched Saturday morning cartoons where *The Superfriends* battled evil, and where Momma Nettie's infamous cheese grits wafted through the air.

Like me, my brother never ventured out to find playmates or to bond with the local kids. A lonesome thinker who sported thick glasses, acne-ridden skin, and an out-of-control afro, my brother kept to himself in the most extreme ways. Being called "Four-eyes," and "Pizza-face," my eleven-year-old brother found relentless harassment from his classmates, which forced him into isolation. Reading mystery books, studying the comic timings of Jerry Lewis, and walking around the house reciting movie speeches aloud, my older brother lost himself in his own world, never relating to others his age.

Besides sharing a last name, my brother and I also shared an isolation that only outcasts could comprehend. So there we were, two persecuted misfits on a couch, indulging in stories that would help us escape from the misery that came with being different.

Moreover than not, heroes presented themselves to me in many ways and, besides the Hulk, another hero careened into my world without warning on a certain Saturday morning. As my brother turned the channels, I saw it on the screen and yelled out, "S-S-S-t-t-top."

The sight of it instantly grabbed me. Its large, scaly figure busted through buildings like a horse through weeds. Its ferocious roar and blazing fire spurted out of its mouth, disintegrating anything in its path. After a moment, my brother wanted to surf the channels again, but I wrestled the remote out of his hands. Even though he had four years on me, my fist carried more experience.

For a half hour I gawked at the misunderstood Godzilla wreaking havoc on Tokyo. When the show ended, I salivated for more, but I'd have to wait till next Saturday. This was before VHS or DVD, where a kid could replay his favorite scenes. But with the help of a pencil and a blank sheet of paper, I could possibly freeze-frame moments from Godzilla's epic battles and relive the grand spectacle that was branded in my head.

In my drawings, planes came from all around. Godzilla trounced on them as fire blazed out of its mouth. Over and over, I drew the scenes until my pencil ran out of lead. Begging Momma Nettie to find me a new sharpened pencil, I raced back to the table and drafted more action-packed pictures.

As the days followed, my hands cramped as I scribbled and jotted on anything I could get my hands on. A cardboard box, a sidewalk with chalk, and the inside on my textbooks fell victim to my artistry. My seven-year-old creations may have been far from Michelangelo's renderings, but I had found something that made me forget about my deficiency. The more sketches I produced, the more normal and less isolated I felt.

Not everyone embraced my craving to sketch. With a terse face, Sister Teresa stared at me from across her desk, "And what do you have to say for yourself? Are you going to continue to keep doing these heathen acts to your books?"

I shook my head. "Is that a yes or a no?" "N-n-n-no m-m-ma'am." I responded.

Flipping through my second grade math textbook, Sister Teresa pointed to a page where Godzilla terrorized math problems. Planes teetered from all around the creature, bombing missiles on plus signs and subtractions. The winged dots looked like gnats, but to me they resembled fighters gliding above the ferocious monster.

"This book is ruined," she said in her thick Irish accent. "What do you have to say for yourself?" Sorrow may have reflected in my face, but my inner confidence carried a different message. I celebrated in my designs as they were displayed in front of the principal. I had created images that would forever be tattooed in a book, and no one could take that away; not the whippings I got from Pop after Momma was called to Sister Teresa's office; not the jeers I experienced from my classmates; and not even my stuttering could rob me of the inner glow I experienced when my pictures came to life. Finally, I felt as if I had something to offer. Without using my mouth, I could communicate.

Regardless of how many times teachers busted me for not paying attention in class, or the other visits I made to Sister Teresa's office, sketching continued to be my hobby of choice. Not only would I recreate stories of an Asian lizard monster, I would also sketch other original creatures that seemed as real as the classmates I saw every day. For hours, I locked myself in my room, translating stories from my thoughts to the pages that were strewn all about me.

Soon I discovered that my newfound art form didn't just cater to my own self-gratification. To show my appreciation for Momma

Nettie, I drew a picture of how I saw my great-grandmother who was beginning to look more sullen and less energetic than before. With long red hair and glowing blue eyes, my version of Momma Nettie had her levitating above our house. She looked youthful as she protected us and watched over our family.

"This is a fine picture," Momma Nettie noted as she raised my drawing high above her. "And I'm looking down at the house, huh?" I nodded.

With the smell of scotch and Salem emanating from her mouth, Momma Nettie kissed me and said, "You know, one day I'll be looking down at ya'll. When I go to heaven, I'll be watching... especially you, baby."

I didn't understand what she meant at the time. None of it made sense. Like a hurdle, I mentally jumped over her comment. Her morbid sentiments had no room for a boy who was just entering his seventh year on earth. All that mattered was that I brought joy to Momma Nettie. Never would she experience my temper or my outbursts again. I would only provide her satisfaction and love through my art. She would forever remain immortal in my drawings.

10 Playing Harpo

"Souls of prayer are souls of great silence."
— Mother Teresa

Almost five years had passed since my Hulkish outburst with Momma Nettie and still, I never attempted to pick up the phone or open the door. When either clanged, I followed my instincts by quietly scampering to my room while someone else answered them.

It was December 1982, and I just turned nine that following November. My silence and sketching kept me isolated from others, so I glided through third grade with no major bumps or bruises. As I entered the fourth grade, my family continually catered to my reluctance by deflecting anything that linked me to the outside world. It was already a given that I wouldn't go near anything ringing or buzzing. I always had a way out. Even when I found myself alone in the living room as Momma Nettie napped, our newly purchased answering machine guarded me from the ringing demon. I was never held accountable, as the coddling had hit an all-time high, and my self-esteem hit an all-time low.

As I caved in from the challenges, a whisper hissed in my head whenever I heard the ringing. *Just answer it. You can do it.* I annoyed myself for such courageous notions. They got me in trouble before, and, most assuredly, they would again.

To block out the self-loathing that came with running away from my fears, I delved even more into my storytelling. Every waking moment was either dedicated to sketching, crayons, or water coloring. My drawing abilities had matured in the last two years. My characters were brave. They were heroes. I tried to see myself in them.

With the help of my brother, I found another medium to forget my ever-looming impediment. On special occasions, when our cousins, grandparents, aunts and uncles gathered at our house for Thanksgiving or Christmas, my brother took full advantage of an already captive audience by performing during family dinners. Acting out scenes from *Smokey and the Bandit* and *Young Frankenstein*, my brother delivered long, outlandish speeches in the same tempo and flair as Jackie Gleason and Gene Wilder.

For his performances, my brother needed someone to appear alongside him in the scenes, a sort of straight man—a fleshy prop—and I was the perfect candidate. While my brother orbited around me delivering punch line after punch line, I stood at the end of the table with him, using facial expressions that bordered on pantomiming. Nothing audible came from my mouth, I left that to the professional. The only direction I got from my brother was to react silently. I was Harpo to his Groucho. We had formed our very own dinner theater. Vaudeville had come to Metairie.

Strangely, I felt at ease with the whole setup. The laughs and the acceptance I felt in the dining room provided an unparalleled thrill. Seeing Momma and Momma Nettie's face turn beet red from laughter, and hearing Pop's unrelenting cackle gave me a satisfaction like no other. Finally, they were laughing with me instead of feeling sorry for me. But soon, the comfort of being a silent performer would hit a dead end, and a tall, husky-voice forty-eight year-old teacher would bring an end to my short-lived serenity.

With almost thirty years under her belt in academia, Ms. Chimento had been St. Benilde's most revered teacher. Similar to how I felt about Ms. Marquez, a sense of comfort waked over me when I was appointed to Ms. Chimento's fourth grade class. Her patience with loud, rowdy students never fazed her or made her lash out. Instead, an authoritarian glare from behind her bifocals made any student shiver with fear. Her magnified gaze was her golden weapon, but she was fair, very fair, and I thought her impartiality would carry over to my stuttering problem.

I would be sorely mistaken.

As Ms. Chimento assigned roles for the annual fourth grade nativity play—which would be performed a week before Christmas in St. Benilde's Church—none of the students, including me, had the courage to share his or her apprehensions in performing. Ms. Chimento's decision was final, never to be questioned or argued. Reading from a list, Ms. Chimento rattled off the names of unfortunate souls who would have to portray the biblical characters. Hovering over my desk, I sketched away, veering my mind elsewhere. I was so immersed in my world of drawings that I didn't hear my name called out.

A nudge from behind and a student's whisper woke me from my solitude, "Hey, that's you."

My eyes darted up as Ms. Chimento's burly figure stood in front of the class. "Are you with us now, Scott?" my teacher asked. Before I could respond, she continued, "Good. So you will be playing Wise Man #1."

I heard a few laughs from around me, and someone grunting under their breath, "I didn't know Wise Men talked like retards."

"That's enough," said Ms. Chimento, who had ears like The Nautilus.

I appreciated her protection, but how could she possibly shelter me from any future calamites, including her own casting choice? By now everyone, including faculty members, knew about the stuttering kid in Chimento's class. I had become tabloid fare, a rumor, and I thought with that said, Ms. Chimento would pass over me in the casting process.

Returning to my sketches, I acted like Ms. Chimento's news didn't disturb me, but, on the contrary, it wrecked me. My insides rattled. The air left my lungs. I felt my morning cereal coming up. *What if I have to say words?* I quietly brooded as my teacher handed out the scripts before the bell rang.

A confused fog filled my head as I made my way back home. What were only a few blocks felt more like a twenty-mile trek. I didn't dare look at the pages that were shoved in my backpack. Since Ms. Chimento handed them out, I couldn't summon enough courage to see if I had any lines. Similar to how I dealt with everything pertaining to stuttering, ignorance was bliss.

Trudging my way home, I allowed my fears to leap from the outrageous to the deranged. I already accepted the fact that I would make a fool of myself in front of the school, but how could I possibly do such a sacrilegious act by stuttering in front of a crucified Christ? Being harangued for sketching in textbooks or for talking funny was one thing, but to be scrutinized and damned by the Almighty in His sacred house was something beyond comprehension. Surely I would be excommunicated from the church and expelled from school. Disgrace would follow me forever. What the hell was I going to do?

I saw Pauley every day in class, yet we hardly spoke with one another. Smiles here, a wave there were the extent of our daily interactions. Sure, I invited him and a couple of kids from school to my Chuck E. Cheese birthday party, where he woofed down a whole pizza by himself, but he and I never truly connected until Ms. Chimento put us together as the two Wise Men. According to Ms. Chimento, we didn't have enough students to fill the shoes for a third magus, so two would have to suffice. Maybe Ms. Chimento believed that Pauley's overweight figure alongside my scrawny body would reflect three magi instead of two.

For years I knew Pauley as the plump kid who gorged by himself and never participated in playground activities. On most days, he hummed random Christmas songs to himself or quoted movies as if someone was always standing next to him. But his unorthodox ways never bothered me like it bothered the other kids. In fact, I took great delight in Pauley's eccentric manners. I was used to it; it felt like home. My brother and I—and my entire family for that matter—were as eccentric as they came. Deep down, I saw myself in Pauley.

Pauley never joined in with the others who picked on me because of my stuttering, and I reciprocated that same respect when it came to his weight. He was an outcast, and because of that we had much in common. Whenever teams were being selected for dodge ball, Pauley and I found ourselves as the last choices. "I guess I'll take fatty, and y'all can take the stutterbird," was the usual remark.

To his credit, Pauley couldn't help it that his body lacked style or grace. It was in his genes. His father had the exact features, which included a hunched over posture, arms dangling to the side, and a set of bowed legs that made his large feet flap with every step. Since kindergarten, Pauley's rotund gut hung over his uniformed pants, earning him gibes and insults like, "Fat-ass," "Titanic," and "Rhino-ass." Because of the barrage of insults, Pauley kept to himself. But unlike me, he dealt with the jeers like Gandhi—smiling, nodding, and walking away to his lonesome corner. It was like he had an impenetrable force field around him, protecting his soul from the ignorant slanders.

The more I hung around Pauley, the more I prayed that my future responses to the smears could mirror Pauley's benevolence. I prayed that I could learn more about the warmhearted kid who loved junk food and people just the same. And I prayed that somewhere in between, God would save me from the role of Wise Man #1. Soon my prayers would be answered in the forthcoming weeks.

The church pew squeaked from under me as I glanced over my script. I couldn't keep still. I squirmed from the unsettling feeling in my gut. In front of the altar, Ms. Chimento positioned the students in various places. Rehearsal had begun and in one week, the altar would be adorned with a manger and cut out sheep and plastic donkeys, and the church would be filled to capacity.

I didn't tell anyone in my family about my performance in the nativity play. To worry them would have caused even more stress to my voice. Besides, my parents were already taking care of Momma Nettie for some ailment that didn't have a name yet. My family had enough on their plate. No, the nativity play was my battle, and I wanted to do it alone.

Looking down, my fears came into fruition as I, for the first time, scanned through my lines for Wise Man #1. Hoping my responsibilities would miraculously disappear, I waited till the last minute to look at the script; perhaps I waited too long. To my dismay, my lines were more than Pauley's.

With a numbness building up on the tips of my fingers, Pauley leaned over my shoulder from the pew behind me and read from my script. I heard Pauley mouth my lines for a few moments. "You got lines, you lucky dog," an exuberant Pauley commented. "That's cool."

I sat there, speechless. Noticing my quiet demeanor, the eight-year old Pauley broke the ice by asking, "You got that thing with your voice, huh?" Looking behind me, I nodded. Pauley had a way with being blunt. He was already picked on by his appearance, what did he have to lose by being honest?

As his stringy hands rubbed over his chin, Pauley came up with the most profound idea, "How about I take your lines?"

My heart leaped out of my chest. My eyes went wide as I stared back at my new best friend. By my reaction, Pauley certainly saw that I was beyond ecstatic. Grabbing the script from my hands, Pauley confirmed that he could do it. He pointed at his new lines and read over them. In his deep, quasi-grown up voice, Pauley gave his best Wise Man voice a whirl, " 'We have traveled far, and now we have come to give Him praise.' "

The thought of saying such words unnerved me, yet Pauley did it beyond perfection. "How was that?" he asked.

"G-G-Good," I replied.

Pauley pointed to my line. Well, actually my word, "Amen."

I mouthed it, but didn't dare say it. With a pat on the back, Pauley assured me that I could do it. *We'll see*, I told myself.

Days later, I felt the polyester robe cling to my body from the nervous sweat dripping from my pores. Pauley led the way as we crossed to the center of the altar. To my left I could see rows of students and faculty members staring on. The choir music stirred from the side of the altar. From where I stood, I saw some of the choir students stretching their necks, reaching for the high notes. *God, I wish I was singing right now.*

Pauley and I hit our mark in front of the plastic baby Jesus. Pauley said his line with meaning and conviction. Then my word came. I was certain if Pauley could do it, then I could do it. All I had to do was open my mouth, take in a deep breath like Hambuga always preached to me, and let it out. Like a Celtic chant, I sang the "A" and then glided into the word. "AAAA-men."

I ignored a couple of whispers in the front row, and I dared not look out into the crowd. My word wasn't perfect, but I said it — well, sang it — and survived. An encouraging smile came from Pauley as he ducked his head away from the congregation and turned a corner of his face toward me.

To this day, I still don't know why Pauley reached out to help me. Was it because he connected with a fellow misfit? Was it because he relished in lines more than I? I still don't know what was behind his saving grace, but the reason didn't matter.

Brandishing a triumphant grin, I looked up at the crucified Christ in front of the altar and prayed. *Thank you, God...for Pauley.*

It was of no coincidence that the first words I uttered in front of an audience meant, "so be it" in Hebrew. Through the word, God gave me the divine right to speak in front of others, and to relinquish my fears, even for a second. He allowed it to be so, and with His allowance, the inaugural step toward my calling had begun.

11 Sherlock Meets Ross

"The invariable mark of wisdom is to see the miraculous in the common."
— *Ralph Waldo Emerson*

In the early months of 1983, an ambiguous confusion intensified within me. Call it the beginning of pubescent hormones escalating, or the exhaustion from a six-year struggle with stuttering thus far—it could've been a mixture of both, but who knows. Whatever the case, I felt deeply alone in a bleak future that awaited me. For sanity's sake, I needed to meet that one person who shared in my affliction, and a chance to exchange similar war stories, anxieties, and miseries. Someone who could offer a sense of kinship and possible relief.

Besides my brother—who I hardly saw since he started high school—Pauley was the only outcast I could somewhat relate with on a daily basis. Films, books, and the latest action figures filled our discussions, yet I wedged my private torments deep within me, never imparting my agonies with anyone, including Pauley who wouldn't understand such issues—or so my ignorance dictated. Perhaps a fellow stutterer could understand and relate to the depths of my despair, but where could I find such a person?

There wasn't a hotline I could just speed dial to locate local stutterers in the area, and asking some random person on the street if he had a speech impediment was too ballsy for an introvert like me. Besides, it was downright weird, especially coming from a stuttering kid.

Determined and desperate, I had to depend on my keen perception to weed out that certain someone. Once I confirmed a stutterer and had all the facts in my favor, perhaps then I could approach the targeted stranger with certainty in my back pocket. Just like I did years prior, studying speech patterns became my tool of choice, but this time I branched out beyond my immediate family.

Since I assumed most stutterers were audibly reserved, I looked for the subtle details when in public: the one-word, stammering answers, and the other coping mechanisms that came with the impediment. During my observations, I picked up on strangers who had slight abnormal vocalizations—a lisp here, a higher register there—but never did I locate a "someone" who stuttered as severely as I did. As I lumbered through those first five months of 1983, my awareness to vocal patterns grew sharper, improved by intense detection. In due time, I became the Sherlock Holmes of articulation.

The first person I deduced as having any semblance to a stutterer came in the form of an outgoing, witty, and charming Sergeant Major. Pop's younger brother didn't come around all that much, but when he did, our household brightened up a little more. On his official leaves from the army, my uncle would mark his arrival by barreling through our front door, while barking in his drill sergeant voice, "Bro-bro-bro...I'm reporting for duty!"

At first I thought his repetition of random words was a funny bit, his charming way of kidding around. Surviving two wars— Vietnam and later, Somalia—my uncle somehow found a way to laugh at life. As the consummate jokester, he always sported a smile, and had a few hearty jokes to tell. To this day I don't ever remember my uncle delving into self-pity or suffering from PTSD. Contrasting with his older brother, my uncle had an innate cheerful disposition that made me laugh. But when he came to visit in March of '83, his repetitious letters and static words affected me on a deeper level. Soon, I realized his supposed stammers didn't stem from his jocular tendencies, but from something else, something undetected by the common ear.

As he and Pop conversed at the dinner table one evening, I overheard my uncle explain how he physically restrained a drunk private, "You see-you see-you see, I tackled this guy and he-he-he he tried to punch back. But I nabbbed-nabbed him right in the stomach."

His quick repeats stuck out. They were similar to my buffers—a tool used to stall time until his mouth caught up with his thoughts. No one had ever labeled my uncle, but I knew a slight stutterer when I heard one.

After much thought, I decided not to engage my uncle with such questions about how he dealt with his stammers. How could I bring up an issue that had never been regarded as an issue? Instead, I studied and admired my uncle from afar. In the process, more farfetched concerns arose in my thoughts: Did I inherit a stuttering pattern from my uncle? Was there a complex, stuttering gene that ran rampant in our family? Unbridled, my young ludicrous assumptions ran rampant.

Another mild stutterer who occasionally dropped by the house was my Pop's best friend from Guatemala. Immigrating to America in the '50s as well, Mr. Frank worked for almost forty years at a local grocery chain as a delivery manager. Sitting out on the porch one afternoon, Mr. Frank and Pop gulped down a few suds. I sat nearby, listening to their stories. As they recalled their tall tales, I couldn't help but study Mr. Frank's vocal patterns, "Now look here...look here, okay...okay, so-so-so I says...I-I-I says, don't do that to the guy."

Though his stutters were a little more severe than my uncle's, Mr. Frank used audible mannerisms that were similar to mine—his sharp, thin lips puttering out repetitious words. Sometimes Mr. Frank's Adam's apple gyrated up and down like a bouncy ball, making a gargling sound as he landed on troubling words. Some would probably presume that Mr. Frank's stammering derived from his difficulty that came when speaking a second language, but the true reasons behind his stammers remain a mystery to me.

I never asked Mr. Frank about his mild impediment or if he had any reservations when he spoke. Doing so would surely be embarrassing to him, or so my guilty conscience assumed. Because of my reservations in not asking these gentlemen about their stammers, deeper questions lingered in my head: If I was so aware of audible quirks, did I subconsciously learn some of my stuttering by passively listening to Mr. Frank and my uncle when I was growing up? Did I pick up on their stammering cadences when they dropped by for visits? Maybe my hidden talent for mimicking became my undoing. Only time would answer such queries.

Needless to say, the opportunity to relate my story with other severe stutterers seemed slim to none. And even if there was a place to congregate for stutterers, where were they located? Like AA meetings, there weren't weekly support groups where stutterers stood up and proudly announced, "H-H-Hi, I-I'm S-Scott and I-I-I'm a st-t-t-tutterer."

"H-H-Hi, S-S-Scott!"

Even if such meetings took place, who would attend? Stutterers cringe at the thought of speaking in front of strangers. And who would come right out and say they were a stutterer in the midst of others? A stutterer's desperate weapon is his solitude, which soon evolves into his purgatory. As the old adage goes: "Shame and silence are hell's playgrounds."

But as fate would have it, on a spring afternoon, when I randomly came across a severe stutterer, hell shrank and purgatory quaked, for I had finally found someone whom I could relate with on an unprecedented level, and who could quash the disgrace that came with stuttering. That certain someone was Ross, and he happened to be the local baker of Metairie

The one thing my brother and I fought over during holidays dinners—besides who was getting seconds of Momma's lasagna— were the bread rolls that garnished our table. Packed with dough and love, those soft, sugary rolls melted in our mouths as we gobbled three or four rolls at a time before the main dish arrived. Every time I bit into one, I wondered who could've designed such a masterpiece. Momma and Momma Nettie hardly baked, so who could have created such morsels?

Driving a few miles into Old Metairie—a downtown area of our suburbs—my eyes gazed out of Momma's Datsun. Just minutes prior, Momma announced that she had to pick up a bag of rolls for our Easter family dinner. I begged her to let me tag along, she reluctantly said yes.

As the historical buildings zipped by, I tried to guess which one housed the magical buns. Parking in front of a random shop, my heart skipped a beat when I read the white letters painted on its front window, "Ross's Bakery." Momma ordered me to stay in the car. Ignoring her, I had already careened out of the car and rushed into the store, where I pressed my hands and face against the glass case to gaze at the muffins, cupcakes, and doughnuts. My eyes went wide at the doughy treasures. Before I had time to take it all in, a man dressed in a white chef uniform peered over the counter. With his baker's hat tilting to the side, he said, "H-H-Hello y-y-young m-m-man. H-H-How are y-y-you?"

His voice shook me at my core. The rolling of his eyes and the gyration of his head sent a shockwave throughout my body. I felt as if I were looking into a mirror. I couldn't say a word; all I could do was stare up at the stuttering baker who sported a welcoming grin. Deflecting my rude gawking, Momma butted in, "Hey, Ross, how are you today?"

"F-F-Fine. A-A-And you, m-m-m-ma'am?"

The self-assurance he exuded blew me away. Showing no signs of humiliation, he didn't care who heard his cacophony of stammers. After his static comments, his face went into a grin; no painful or apprehensive expression followed. He had a business to run, and a life to live. Ross made stuttering look and sound so...normal.

"B-B-Be with you i-i-in a m-m-moment," Ross said to another customer who had just made his way into the bakery.

Wrapping my mind around the fact that a stutterer actually spoke without shame, without hesitation, and with a smile was nearly impossible to comprehend. All I could do was stare at Ross as if he were the 8th Wonder of the World. Again, Momma took notice at my unceasing glare, and with a backhand slap on the arm, whispered, "Don't stare. Don't be rude."

I couldn't help myself. I had found him, and I didn't care how rude I came across, or about other trivial matters, like the rolls or how many doughnuts Momma would buy for tomorrow's breakfast. All I thought about was the courage that the baker exuded. I wanted to prop up on a stool and watch Ross in his natural habitat for the rest of the day while he greeted customers, answered phones, and asked if someone wanted a sample. But eventually, we had to leave, and it took a tight tug from Momma to get me out of the bakery.

On our way home, Momma asked if I was okay. By my quiet demeanor, she probably assumed that I was upset by Ross's stuttering. Perhaps that was the reason she told me to stay in the car. Maybe she didn't want me to see someone else in a similar dilemma.

Turning to Momma, I said, "O-O-One, d-d-day, I-I-I want t-t-to...um...b-b-be like R-R-um, um, Ross."

Taken aback by my comment, Momma asked with a curious glint in her eyes, "You mean, you want to be a baker?"

I shook my head. "I-I-I w-want to b-b-um-b-be normal."

But I was wrong; Ross didn't even come close to being normal. He was exceptional because he never felt sorry for himself, and never let his dysfunction get in the way of his vibrant personality. Like Ross, if I embraced my dysfunction and my imperfections, then maybe, just maybe I could finally taste my future potential.

So many times after my first encounter with Ross, I wanted to return to the bakery and ask him how he dealt with his stuttering, yet my timidity took over. To this day, I regret not bombarding him with questions. But what would I have asked? What could I have said? No, Ross's actions spoke louder than any wisdom he could've imparted to me. His influence and unforgettable example was what I carried with me for years to come, and they filled me more than his rolls.

Ross didn't know it, but by his display of fearlessness, he unleashed a plan that had been simmering in the back of my mind, a plan that lay dormant and stagnant in the crevices of my fears. Soon I would introduce Pauley to this plan. I was ready take charge and not let fear dictate my future because a humble baker inspired me to do so.

12 A Cast of Outcasts

"Anybody who goes to the theater, I think we're all misfits, so we ended up on stage or in the audience."
— Patti LaPone

In front of Pauley, I unrolled the poster that I had labored over for the past week. Proudly, I gestured to it and asked his thoughts about the name of our newly formed group. Staring at the letters that sparkled in gold and red glitter, Pauley mouthed the words on the poster, "Theeee Moooovieeee Plaaaayerrrrs."

Crossing my arms, I studied Pauley's reaction, hoping for a hint of enthusiasm from him, a similar enthusiasm that had been roaring inside of me for some time. Ever since my love for storytelling became an obsession, the urge to act out movies in a safe environment had been pestering me to no end; and by a safe environment I meant a locked room where no audience was allowed and no critical eyes could judge my damaged voice. Hence, the idea to form a club came into play, a group where fellow lovers of cinema could reenact our favorite movies. I wanted to taste, feel, and speak the scenarios that were larger than life, larger than my suburban world, yet I couldn't accomplish this alone.

My long awaited idea was not only ignited by Ross, or when I silently performed alongside my brother during family dinners. Four years prior, my concept was just a silly notion that fermented in my head while spending countless hours studying films in the vastness of a movie theater. This was before cable and HBO invaded living rooms, and the only way to see movies in 1979 was to actually go to the theater.

I had just turned six, and my brother was ten. To get us out of her hair, Momma ordered my brother to take me to the movies at a local movie house. After Momma gave us a few dollars for tickets, Coke, and popcorn, we sped the ten blocks to the cinema. Sitting in the midst of stale popcorn, sticky floors, and gum-stained cushioned seats, we glued our attention to the screen.

Because he took a liking to our constant patronage and the excitement we exuded every time we entered his theater, the owner allowed us to watch the featured film three or four times in a row, and it didn't take long before we knew the films almost verbatim. During those Saturday afternoons, nothing else existed except the darkness surrounding me, the story that unfolded on the screen, and the invincibility I found in the characters. Flash Gordon and James Bond snuck their way into my imagination, for they represented who I wanted to be—a hero, a perpetual figure of perfection. To capture this perfection, I mouthed the lines in unison with them.

I'd repeat the dialogue in their cadence, "Shaken, not stirred," "Bond, James Bond." The movie theater became my sacred temple, my church, my holy of holies.

Peering over my knees as my arms tightly bound around my legs, I took in every line, every quote like a junky on crack. It would take my brother nudging me a few times to stop me from repeating the lines out loud. When I said words in concert with those illuminated faces, I didn't stutter. Their inflections were my inflections. Their adventures became my adventures. I lost myself in their heroic struggles. Thus, this unprecedented and euphoric connection inspired my grand plan.

I never thought it was possible to form a players group with someone else. Who in their right mind would want to join in such a venture with a stutterer? It seemed absurd and full of contradictions, like a blind man forming an archery club. So I filed the idea into my category of impossibilities, never allowing it to blossom into fruition.

But all that changed when I forged a friendship with Pauley. Towards the end of fourth grade, Pauley and I grew closer, like two peas in a pod. We'd spent many Saturdays hooping and hollering at the car chases and shootouts in the movie theaters. As captivated as we were by those images that flickered before us, I decided I wanted to experience my favorite stories in a more vivid and intimate setting.

Staring at "The Movie Players" poster for a few minutes, Pauley still didn't say a word. I thought maybe he needed some convincing, "A-A-After w-w-we see the m-m-um, um, m-movie, then w-w-we c-c-can um c-come b-b-back and act out the m-m-movie here."

My arms extended out, further explaining how my room could be our soundstage, and how we could even dress up like our favorite characters. I pointed out how my bed could be Bond's Aston Martin. A plastic plate could substitute for Tron's discus.

Catching on, Pauley gave me the smile I had been waiting for. He was hooked. We both signed the poster and agreed to tape it on my locked door whenever our "productions" were in session.

We wasted no time bringing "The Movie Players" into existence. Rushing to the cinema almost every day that summer, we plopped down in the last row of the theater and studied the movies like film critics, dissecting scenes and wondering what parts we would play. Soon I introduced my notepad into the mix. With the aid of a flashlight, I took extensive notes containing plot points that would be essential for our reenactments.

Return of the Jedi, Jaws 3-D and *Octopussy* were just some of the movies we watched with keen eyes and careful note taking. After viewing the movies more than once, we charged back to my house, threw on crude costumes, and performed the movie from beginning to end. Sometimes I'd play the bad guy, other times Pauley took on the role of the adversary. We rotated in and out of characters like schizophrenic patients. Even though the stammering was evident in my impromptu dialogue, I was in my glory.

As our friendship evolved, I grew more comfortable stammering in front of Pauley. He paid no mind to my stutters, even when I sounded like a backed up muffler. Reciprocally, I paid no mind to his awkward body movements as he dove from imaginary bullets. When we played in our phantom world of heroes and world-dominating bad guys, we embodied perfection and acceptance, as we brought out the best in one another.

Then the mother lode came; like manna from heaven, Pauley's parents bought a laserdisc player, where we could watch movies on disks in the privacy of Pauley's home. No longer did we have to trek to the movie theaters, take notes, or paraphrase dialogue. We felt like gods of cinema.

Thanks to his father's love for action films, Pauley's collection of James Bond movie disks multiplied in two weeks. Now we had the king of espionage at our fingertips. Day and night, during many sleepovers, we locked ourselves in Pauley's room, watching Sean Connery and Roger Moore battle it out with international villains. By just pressing play, we were teleported to Morocco, London, and the Nile. Being able to pause, rewind, and replay, we had the luxury to master the accents of the characters we wanted to recreate. Repetitively, I'd listen to their tones and cadences. With my compulsive side taking over, I'd play back one line of dialogue ten to twenty times, mouthing the foreign pitches. Little did I know, my fascination with accents would lead to something so unpredictable and so miraculous that it would exceed anything I could have ever imagined.

After studying Dr. No's accent for a half hour, I took my best shot at the infamous villain for one of our reenactments. Playing the role of James Bond, Pauley stood on the other side of his room. Brandishing a ruler that mimicked a Walter PPK, I pointed the twelve inches toward Pauley.

I quoted Dr. No's line from the movie with my best attempt at a British accent, "You're mine, Mr. Bond."

It was a short line—four words—but to my astonishment, they glided out of me. For the first time, my stutter fell to the wayside when I recalled a line with a dialect. No more did I have to say the words with the actor to achieve fluency, I held it on my own. This surprised not only me, but Pauley as well, who gawked at me, speechless.

Like a music prodigy who listens to a song and then plays the exact chords on a piano, I had acquired a similar talent for hearing accents and imitating them. By listening to a dialect a few times, I could then manipulate my mouth to mirror the tone in a fluent delivery. But how did I achieve this elocution? And why did this anomaly occur only with accents?

There were several reasons.

The rewiring of my voice lessened the self-awareness and shame that came with my usual speaking voice. Similar to singing, the right side of my brain instantly took over when I delivered dialects, guiding me past my bad no-no's and my self-sabotaging ways. All I had to do was forget myself and vocally become someone else, and my elocution followed. Also, when delivering the accents, I placed my tongue in different positions than my normal placements, which also lent to my elocution.

According to Hollywood legend, I wasn't the only stutterer who benefited from this voice-manipulation technique. Known as a closet stutterer (aren't we all), Marylyn Monroe mastered a breathy voice that eliminated her stuttering. Some thought her tone was natural, an innate part of her sensuality, but in retrospect, her signature voice was produced consciously; a coping technique that led to a sexy reputation and a prosperous stutter-free career. Later, I would follow Marilyn's strategy by utilizing different voice modulations to hide my stuttering in my theatrical pursuits. But that would be many years later, and a mere glimmer of possibilities in the back of a nine-year old's mind. For now, the usage of accents was a desperate attempt at fluency, and I took full advantage of it.

Outside of our "Movie Players," I started communicating in different dialects while at home. Even if my accents sounded Irish mixed with Russian, I found relief in my new tactic. Like singing, my family allowed me to use funny voices in the house. More than anything, I wanted to answer the phone in an accent, but I had to restrain myself. The caller would probably think they had the wrong number and hang up. Knowing my parents, they wouldn't tolerate such an obnoxious occurrence to happen in their house, especially when Pop had business calls coming in.

My family didn't place too much optimism in my fluency with dialects because we all knew what the inevitable entailed. Sooner or later, in the outside world, I wouldn't be able to use my collection of artificial voices — reality had no room for my playful crutch. But until I was forced to use my normal voice, I spoke in my accents with fanfare.

Sadness filled my heart as our summer days of '83 came to a close. Pauley and I would go our separate ways. The former continued on to the fifth grade at St. Benilde, while I would follow in my brother's footsteps, and attend a prep school that would challenge my fragile personality. With growing up and going to different schools, losing friends along the way was part of the game. It was an unfair side of life for a kid who found making friends just as difficult as speaking. And so, as fall approached, our "Movie Players" had come to an end.

But the distance in time and space never devalued my fondness for Pauley, and how, together, we found a common voice. On those summer days of play-acting and heroic reenactments, we broke free of the names that others branded us. Through our limitless imagination, we had a glimpse of our true selves by becoming other people.

Armed with just the memory of Pauley, I would soon venture alone, relying on my survival skills in a school that brought about the most embarrassing event to ever happen to me.

13 The Wet Evidence

"Warriors should suffer their pain silently."
— Erin Hunter, Into the Wild

My eyes danced around, taking in the wonderment of it all—its high ceilings, gothic-gated entryway, and the marble floors and walls with their milky, smooth finish. For a moment, the school swept me into a literary world, something out of a thriller where the killer's shoes would echo down the corridors while chasing his next victim.

Beyond the *Jack The Ripper* scene that jogged through my mind and the mansion-turned-prep-school that surrounded me, an excitement pounded in my chest. Each step I took toward my first day of class stomped out the distant memory of St. Benilde—the name-calling, the scarlet letter that had followed me around since first grade, and the loneliness. Amid my new surroundings, I had a new lease on life and a new reputation to forge.

Christian Brothers Academy was the name of my beacon of hope. Founded by the order of the same name, this all boys school—that was once John Audubon's mansion in the 19th Century—had a waiting list a mile long. Having an illustrious reputation for almost sixty years, Christian Brothers was where most of the predominate politicians, lawyers, and doctors in New Orleans sent their kids for grooming, which would inevitably lead to any high school of their choosing. How and why I got accepted into the elite school baffled me. I guess my grades and the recommendations from Ms. Marquez and Ms. Chimento were more laudatory than I thought. Either way, I was playing with the big boys now.

My blue-collar background contrasted with most of the students who rushed past me, making their way to class. I caught site of the students' latest fashions—Polo shirts, Bass shoes and alligator belts. My family's budget had no room for fifty-dollar pairs of shoes and hundred dollar slacks. My sensible parents invested more on higher education and less on fashion, so I wore K-Mart loafers, a shirt with an insignia that looked more like a drunken bandito on a mule than a polo player, and a pair of slacks that resembled brown curtains. A victim to my parents' practicalities, I felt like an outsider already.

Sitting in my designated seat, I scanned the classroom. The thirty students around me created a stir. Talking and laughing, they probably knew each other from former schools. Contrastingly, I remained quiet as I devised a plan on how to be one of the cool kids. Maybe using a different accent would help—a Western twang, or an English accent could prove viable. I could pretend I moved from some far off place—Wales, Liverpool, New Mexico, or anywhere. One problem remained, though. If I did follow such a strategy, I would have to continue my deception until I graduated in three years. Lies upon lies would stack on top of one another, and nothing worthwhile could ever come from keeping this sham at play.

Besides, my brother had done something similar; he hatched his own degree of deceptions, and that didn't pan out well for him. Four years prior to my arrival at Christian Brothers, my brother attended the same school and barely graduated. Still being the spiteful loner, my brother didn't apply himself. He had other priorities to focus on, like spreading rumors that Johnny Carson was his great-uncle, and that a Broadway contract awaited him after graduation. According to my brother's morality scale, superfluous attention outweighed the importance of higher grades. In class, the teachers would bust him practicing his signature in textbooks and on worksheets. When the teachers demanded an explanation, my brother replied, "I have to make sure my signature looks good so I'll know how to sign my photos when I become famous."

So far, our family's name didn't really stand out at Christian Brothers, and I felt my family's reputation weighing heavily upon my shoulders. I was on rebound duty for better grades, no lies, and no sketching in textbooks. Being the better son and student, I wanted to please my family to no end, and pleasing them was one of my top priorities. Even if I wanted to forget my responsibilities, I had Pop reminding me religiously, "Don't screw up like your brother. We paid a lotta goddamn money for you to go to that school. You want to work under cars for the rest of your life like me?"

I took his attempt at a pep talk to heart, and I was ready to apply myself. My commitment would not only impress my family, but would impress others, especially Christian Brothers' faculty and the new students who sat around me. I didn't want to be the problem child.

On that first day of school when butterflies smacked around my stomach and my adrenaline pumped like an oil rig, I almost jumped out of my seat when the French doors swung open and in came a bald-headed scholar who looked more like a Shakespearean actor than a fifth-grade teacher. Students shifted in their seats as the teacher bee-lined to the front of the class. His intense eyes scanned the room as he went to the board and wrote, "My name is Brother Raphael" — fourteen letters of a name that would change the world as I knew it.

During those first weeks of school, my nights were dedicated to grueling homework assignments. Some of those late hours were spent at the kitchen table with Pop helping me with science, my most troubling class. After taking the recent biology pop quizzes, my scores were less than impressive. In order to better my grades, Pop and I stayed up late into the night, repeating over and over the particulars about cells, nuclei, and symbiosis. To me, they sounded like sci-fi characters. Out of boredom I'd stare off and daydream about how they appeared in my galactic world — slimy arms, five heads, and bulging eyes. My ray gun blasted them as I saved Earth. *Take that Evil Symbiosis!*

Slapping the back of my head, Pop scolded me, "Pay attention, son! You have to apply yourself!"

If I flunked one more science test, Pop would take a belt to my ass for sure. But he was right. I had to stay focused, keep quiet, make A's, and don't let anyone know of my secret. That was my long-term plan.

Three weeks into the fifth grade, my stratagem took a turn for the worse when Brother Raphael announced our next assignment, "Today, lads, each of you will take turns and read portions of this book out loud."

His announcement hit me like a steamroller. *Not again*, I thought. I was dizzy. I couldn't breathe. I didn't know what to do.

"I want to hear each student read out loud from this book." Raphael held the book above his head, as if he were showing an evangelical congregation the Good News. The title read, "The Most Dangerous Game." *How appropriate*, I thought.

"Classics deserve their respect, and you, lads, must learn this. Enunciation with literature is everything," stated Brother Raphael, as he walked to his desk at the front of class. "Now, if I hear a mistake, I will stop and correct you." His words punched out with an intimidating resonance, like they always did.

I looked around to see if any of the other boys shared in my terror. All the students wore the same look of disinterest about the lesson as they reluctantly flipped open their books. Christ, I would have given anything to be as disinterested as everyone else, instead of being scared shitless.

"When I tap the pen on my desk, one student will begin reading where the other one left off…and so on, and so on," Raphael said, pointing forward. "We will start with the first row and go on down."

First row? My row. My heart skipped a beat as I counted the students before me. Just like Ms. Marquez's class, three students sat between the inevitable nightmare and me. Giving up my secret would not only flunk me out of English, but would force Pop into punishing me for the rest of my life. I had already predicted my fatal outcome. I was trapped in my own horror version of déjà vu.

CLICK! CLICK! CLICK!

Brother Raphael's silver Cross-pen banged on his desk. It sounded like a courtroom gavel, and I was about to be prosecuted by an unforgiving jury. With a whisper to his voice, Andrew Albright, the first student in my row, began to read.

"Louder, Mr. Albright," shouted Raphael as his deep resounding voice filled the classroom.

Following orders, Andrew yelled out every word as if the class was trapped in a wind tunnel. A few snickers came from the students. I covered my ears and hummed gently to myself. *They're going to laugh more at me.*

CLICK! CLICK! CLICK!

Raphael's pen knocked again. It echoed like a gunshot. My eyes popped wide open as I stared forward. My turn was coming up and there was nothing I could do to stop it. Or maybe there was, maybe I could go to the bathroom again. But how long would that ruse last? Sooner or later, Raphael would catch on. He was smarter than any other teacher I had encountered, and he wouldn't buy into such ploys.

The second student in my row started reading. He enunciated each word like poetry. I looked up at the fluorescent lights vibrating and pulsing in their tubes. I reflected on Ms. Hambuga's lessons from years prior, "Sing the vowels and connect the consonants." In my head, I quietly hummed vowels over and over again. It was my only rope to hold onto as I sank further into the quagmire of self-doubt.

CLICK! CLICK! CLICK!

Right in front of me, Mickey Carlson took his turn at reading aloud. *Holy Jesus, I'm next.* Sweat flowed down my sides. My hands turned clammy. My head was about to explode from the stress. There was so much pressure in my head that I was on the verge of passing out. I needed a distraction, any distraction from this volcanic fear bubbling up inside of me.

My eyes wandered away from the book and onto Brother Raphael. Like a halo, his baldhead gleamed from the overhead lights, as he sat upright at his desk. He had an angelic elegance about him. Perhaps it was his neatly trimmed goatee, or the way his head and neck remained unbent as he glared down at his book. *Like Zeus looking down on his mere mortals,* I thought in wonderment.

Suddenly, I recited a silent prayer: *Please, Brother, look at this mortal. Stop the class. Take me outside. Save me from all this, before I...*

CLICK! CLICK! CLICK!

I froze. Looking down, I caught the first word of the paragraph I was supposed to read, "There." T-h...one of my bad no-no's. My tongue pressed against the inside of my teeth as spit shot out. I tried to release that first word, but instead my mouth resembled a sprinkler.

"Mr. Damian, you're next," ordered Raphael.

I know! I wanted to yell out, but my mouth didn't open. It clenched down, as if an invisible hand held my jaw shut. Everything in my body went tight as the shakes worsened. Then it came; an accent that I had stored in the recesses of my memory and suddenly released without thinking. The dialect was slightly English with a touch of Cockney. Without a doubt, the accent stemmed from one of the Bond movies. My desperation had shoved it out. I had to say something, anything to fill the void.

In my invented voice, the first sentence came out of my mouth, "There is no greater bore than perfection." My eyes gaped wide open as relief quenched my heated anxiety. I continued on in my quasi-British accent. Laughs roused around me. I didn't know if they were laughing at me, or just getting a kick out of my rendition of Dr. No reading a classic.

"Stop!" yelled Brother Raphael as his deep timber bounced off the walls.

Time stood still. The voice of Zeus had spoken. Noticing a change in Raphael's tone, I anticipated his next words to be one of praise for my glorious enunciation.

Sliding off his glasses, Raphael leaned forward, "Are you trying to patronize this assignment, young man?"

Holding my breath, I couldn't think of a response.

"Are you like your brother...insolent and can't take directions without making a mockery of my class?"

Earnestly, I tried to explain myself to my new teacher. "N-N-N-No, th-th-th-th..."

"Speak up, young man. I can't understand what you're saying."

Looking down at my book, I wanted to make it right as I tried to read in my normal voice, but my throat locked. Not a word was coming out as I pushed harder. My methodical symptoms came out in all their glory—the shaking of the head, and the gurgling sound beating from the back of my mouth. My anxiety, embarrassment, and shame had hit a crescendo.

A discord of laughs burst around me. They weren't laughing with me anymore, they were now laughing *at* me. Suddenly, like opening a shaken Coke bottle, a release exploded from my body, just below my pleather belt.

Guffawing an obnoxious laugh, Mickey turned around. Instantly, he stopped laughing as something caught his attention. He glanced down. His hand flew up, motioning for Brother Raphael to come near.

"Mr. Carlson, what is it now?" asked Brother as he raised himself up from his throne behind the desk and headed toward Mickey and me. All the heads in the classroom followed the mystery that was occurring in the back of the class. I wanted to tell Mickey to turn around, but I couldn't move. I couldn't even speak. The shock of it all paralyzed me.

As Brother neared us, Mickey lowered his hand and pointed down. Behind his thick black-rimmed glasses, Raphael's eyes locked on where Carlson was pointing. A puddle of urine had formed below my desk. Through my pants and down my K-Mart loafers, the yellow trickled down like a waterfall.

"Brother," Mickey said with a smile. "I think he pissed his pants."

More uproarious laughter echoed throughout the room. The amused eyes witnessed the wet evidence of my uncontrollable fears. I placed my hands over my ears, trying to stop the cruel laughter. But nothing could silence the concern that settled in my broken heart: What would my parents think of their son now?

14 Life Ain't Cheap

"Life is a fight, but not everyone's a fighter. Otherwise, bullies would be an endangered species."
— Andrew Vachss

Angels appear in places of obscurity, in the trenches of life when harsh realities whisk by you like bullets from a muzzle, when you're about to give up, and when all hope is lost. Crawling through my trenches on that devastating day, I stumbled upon an angel and, to my surprise, he was a helluva a lot better than Zeus.

As soon as he realized what I had done to myself, Brother Raphael rushed me out of class, threw my soiled pants into the washing machine and replaced them with a pair of sweats.

"How are you holding up, lad?" asked a gentler Brother Raphael as I tried to compose myself in a corner of the library.

I didn't respond to Brother's question at first. Embarrassed by my unrelenting tears, I quickly wiped my cheeks and rubbed my hands on my oversized sweat pants. I hated crying in front of others, it showed too much of my fragility. In addition to the crying and the stuttering, the disgrace that came with pissing on myself made me want to burrow under a rock for the next ten years. I wondered if Ross ever experienced anything like this. *Probably not.*

Sensitive to my distraught state, Brother Raphael profusely apologized, saying he didn't know of my stutter. For the rest of the day, my teacher allowed me to stay in the library, away from the other students. Trying to offer me some form of comfort, Raphael explained how he would speak to the class, and that my situation could've happened to anyone.

"There is no reason to feel ashamed," he reiterated.

Before he left, I desperately pleaded with Brother Raphael, begging him not to mention the incident to my parents. After much coercion, Brother agreed, but not without adding his words to the unwise, "Lad, this will pass. I promise. Don't let this dictate your worth and who you will become."

By the intensity on his face, I could tell Brother Raphael had been through something similar. Veterans of pain can detect fellow veterans. To this day, I don't know all the particulars behind Brother Raphael. All I know is that something lingered behind Brother's blue eyes like an open-ended conclusion.

Glancing up at my teacher, I gave him my first smile of the day. Supplying me with a candy bar, a soda pop, and a pat on the head, Brother Raphael returned to class, leaving me among a parade of books. In that library, a mutual bond was formed between Brother Raphael and me and as a result, a trust was born. Thus, my long love for the sixty-something year old Brother had begun.

No matter how hard he tried, nothing in Brother Raphael's bag of influential dictums could protect me from the slanderous eyes and unrelenting names that would come my way in the weeks and months that followed. Similar to my stay at St. Benilde, names like "Freak," "Stutterbird," and the new, ever-so-popular "Soily Scott" bombarded me as I went about my days at Christian Brothers. Shoves and snickers behind my back were common occurrences. My new lease on life was revoked as news of my wet incident ran rampant throughout the school. Some students claimed that I came from a Special-Ed home. Another speculation alleged that I had a partial lobotomy. One rumor vouched that my parents were actually brother and sister, and I was their deformed product.

Without any options, I allowed the rumors and the sneers to roll off my shoulders; I guess Pauley's Gandhi approach had influenced me more than I realized. I kept my nose in the books and remained quiet. Committed to my well being, Brother Raphael checked in with me on a daily basis. "How are you lad?" was the question he always asked me before and after classes. They were the only kind words I'd hear throughout the day.

Like prison, I waited out my time at Christian Brothers. Whenever Momma picked me up and asked about my day, I'd force a bright smile, and say, "F-F-Fine." I didn't want my family to worry about my incessant sadness, and I didn't want to bring coddling and anxiety back into the home again. My parents needed to focus more on Momma Nettie who, for the most part, was in and out of hospitals.

For all Momma assumed, her little man had adjusted to his new environment. For all Momma Nettie knew, her "bust 'em up" was thriving beyond his impediment. For Pop, my days of academic excellence were pushing onward, at least better than my brother's. Keeping secrets from my loved ones had evolved into an acquired talent. But there was one incident I couldn't keep in the dark for too long; an incident I would later call "The Johnny Finger Incident."

The son of a dentist, and one of the richest kids at the academy, Johnny Finger had no comprehension of what boundaries meant. If Johnny wanted it, he got it. The silver spoon he was born with reminded him and everyone around him that he had nothing to pay for, nothing to work for, and no one to answer to. Prancing around and showing off his new tape player and his latest Nike sneakers gave him status. With his entitlement, he pushed the limits, earning his reputation as "The Finger." Actually, his real name wasn't Finger. He earned the illustrious name by raising his middle finger high in the sky and pointing it behind Brother Raphael's back as the latter scribbled on the chalkboard. The giggles that encouraged Johnny to do such a crude act to my protector churned an unforgiving furor within me. But as a silent witness, there was nothing I could do. Helplessly slumped in my desk, I looked on as Finger relished in his prominence, just like he celebrated in the daily slurs and the physical abuses he flung my way.

Tackling me behind the basketball court became a weekly occurrence for Johnny and his gang. Johnny would sit on my chest as two of his cronies held my hands and feet down.

"Whatcha gonna do now, stutterbird, piss in your pants again?" Johnny would ask.

Squirming and shaking under Finger, claustrophobia hit me in the worst way. As much as I tried to writhe my way free, the three boys overpowered me. All I could do was accept the inevitable—Johnny spitting in my face, licking his fingers, sticking them in my ears, and plowing hard blows into my midsection.

"You give me dirty looks in class!" Johnny said as he jabbed at my body between his taunts. "You look like you wanna hit me." PUNCH! "You can't even talk." PUNCH! "How are you going to hit me?" PUNCH!

Everything in me wanted to tell Brother Raphael about Finger's masochistic behavior, but I restrained myself. If I told Brother, then most assuredly, Johnny would seek out revenge. If I told Momma or Pop, the principal would get involved. And I couldn't let Momma Nettie know of my constant harassment. She was already dealing with her own problems, and more stress would add more complications to her mysterious illness. No, I had to keep the peace and remain the good boy.

As much as I tried, I could only sustain the good boy facade for so long. Pushed and prodded enough, I would eventually relinquish the ruse and stand up for myself. I may not have invited him, but the Hulk came for a visit on an unforgettable day, where the details still reside heavily in my thoughts, almost thirty years later.

The Friday afternoon school bell rang, and I raced out of class to the designated pickup area. Every afternoon Momma picked me up in front of the pond in her new ruby-red Malibu Classic.

An unsettling feeling overcame me on this particular afternoon. My head tilted back and forth, trying to see a glimpse of her car. Similar to how I anticipated a bad no-no creeping up and strangling my throat, I sensed an air of hostility surrounding me, forcing its ominous fingers upon my shoulders. I felt it under my skin. I turned, but there was no one, just the trees and the scent of algae floating off the pond.

Relieved, I leaned on a tree and glanced down at my scratched Mickey Mouse watch: 3:40. *Where's Momma?* I wondered. She was usually never this late. All around me, kids barreled into Jaguars, BMW's, and Porches. With their parents behind the wheel, most of my peers were whisked away to a much-anticipated Spring Break, which probably included beachfront homes, warm sand, and amusement parks. I had a different fate awaiting me. My break entailed sweating over countless tire rotations, oil changes, and laborious twelve-hour days in Pop's auto shop. But Pop insisted that my brother and I help out during our break.

Frequently, he would remind us, "You want to go to the best school? Well, you're going to have to work hard for it. Life ain't cheap. A man has to pay a price to get what he wants."

As I reflected on the grueling days that awaited me, I felt a sting from the sudden slap on my shoulder. I knew the grip. I knew the feel of the hand. I knew the face looking down at me as I spun around.

"Heya, stutterbird, where ya been?" asked Johnny Finger. "Were you hiding from me?"

I could've sworn Johnny was gone, that his limo had already glided in front of the school to pick up his wise ass. I hated being wrong. Shutting my eyes, I wanted to disappear. I wanted to hide. I wanted Momma to pull up and save me.

Like two massive pillars, Matthew and Georgie Walter, twins, stood next to Johnny — the same goons who always held down my wrists and feet, and who followed Johnny around like lost sheep. Pointing at my shoes, Matthew scowled, "Don't you look pretty in them cheap shoes. I bet your Mom picked them out for you, didn't she? Didn't that old bag?"

"D-D-Don't say n-n-n-nothing ab-b-bout my M-M-Momma," I snapped back.

They laughed in unison at my feeble attempt to defend Momma. Johnny stepped in closer. The scent of his steamy breath repulsed me. My stomach churned from his foul smell.

"Hey guys, lookie here," said Johnny. "I think Scotty here is gonna to piss in his pants again. Watch out, he needs some room to get the piss out!"

Cackling out loud, Matthew and Georgie high-fived each other. Johnny leaned into my ear, and whispered, "W-W-W-What's the m-m-m-matter stut-t-t-terbird? C-C-Can't t-t-talk?"

I closed my eyes. My body went tight. I knew what was coming next. Johnny cocked his arm back. His fist came straight down and hammered into my shoulder. It felt like a meat cleaver slicing into me. I bit down on my lower lip, to the point of making it bleed. My face turned away from Johnny. I couldn't let him have the satisfaction in knowing that I was dizzy with pain.

I heard Johnny make a guttural, scratchy sound in his throat. It was a hacking sound I had heard a few times before when Johnny straddled me on the basketball courts. Summoning up a ball of mucus, Johnny puckered his lips and projected a thick glob of saliva that splattered onto my face. I felt it drip off my forehead. Tears welled up in my eyes.

Johnny looked me up and down like a predator assessing his prey. He shook his head and began to laugh, "You're gonna piss in your pants, ain't you? Didn't your mom go buy you diapers?" He snapped his fingers in the air, acting as if he was correcting himself, "Oh, that's right, that bitch can't buy nothing. Your mom's corner is slow these days." He snickered at me, turned and slowly walked away.

Everything around me became hazy — the cars, the tree next to me, even the Walter twins. The only thing that remained in focus was Johnny Finger and his enormous back. My whole body shook; not out of nervousness, but from something I had never shown outside of my home — wrath, complete and utter wrath.

I didn't think. Instinct took over as I charged toward Johnny like a bull out of a pen. My fist rose up and over my head. Matthew was the first to see me, "Johnny, look out!"

But it was too late. All Johnny could do was turn and face the inevitable. My knuckles connected to Johnny's left brow with a force that threw the much larger ten-year old onto his back. His cranium felt harder than our walls back home, but the adrenaline pumping through my body didn't give me the satisfaction to feel the burn on my knuckles.

I jumped on Johnny and, like a windmill in a hurricane, my fists rotated down onto his face. Georgie placed his hand on my arm, but I came in with a backhand roundhouse that snapped him in the jaw. Instantly, Georgie went down. Matthew grabbed both my arms from behind me. I pushed his arms off of me and elbowed him hard in the face. I felt his nose crack on the point of my elbow. Matthew fell over like a broken tree.

I climbed back on Johnny and continued my relentless assault. Hit after hit sliced into Johnny. His hands waved around, a feeble attempt to protect his face. But there was nothing he could do; I had him, and I wasn't going to let him go. The anger was too deep. The rage was too much. I had been a good boy for too long.

A deluge of defeats, suffering, and shame came pouring down on Finger. I had lost control. I wasn't punching Finger anymore. I was impaling every hurtful word that passed through my ears. I was hitting against God, who gave me such a cross to bear. I was striking down on all those who laughed, jeered, and looked at Pauley, Ross, and me with critical eyes.

Snapping out of my state of possession, the color of ruby-red caught my attention. I looked up. A few yards away, I saw Momma's Malibu Classic. Through the windshield, her face leaned forward as her chin rested on the steering wheel. I scanned around and witnessed onlookers glaring at me. The temper subsided as the reality of the situation became clearer.

Like erasing any evidence of guilt, I wiped Johnny's blood and saliva from off my face with my sleeve. As I picked up my backpack, I dashed toward the car. A whimper came from Johnny as he turned to his side, holding his nose and mouth. The drumbeat sound of the muffler welcomed me as I opened the passenger door. I plopped down on the seat, and set my backpack on the floor. The smell of grass, mud, and sweat drifted from my body into the perfume-scented car.

Momma faced me with a concerned look. Humiliated and ashamed, I glanced down. I stared at my hands, which were covered with red splotches. The aches from the jabs were settling into my knuckles. "P-P-Please d-d-don't tell Pop." I pleaded. "I-I-I'm s-s-s-sor-r-ry, M-M-Momma. Th-Th-Th-They said th-th-things ab-b-b-bout you…"

She placed her soft hands on my red, dirt-smeared face, "They make you fight. I know that," whispered Momma, "because you're different. They're gonna to make you fight."

Sliding over, she wrapped her arms around my dirty neck and leaned into me. I felt her tears on my face. Her cheek pressed against my sore shoulder, yet my shoulder didn't hurt as much as before.

"Sometimes a man has to fight his own battles…alone." Momma whispered. "You're a man. My baby is a man now."

Her words warmed over me like a blanket during winter. I realized I didn't need some exotic beach, a high-priced trip, or expensive shoes to make me feel whole. All I needed was the woman whose honor I defended to call me a man. That was enough for me. That was my affirmation—my baptism.

Momma continued to rub my back as my head rested in her arms. Through my tears, I stared out the car window. In the distance, I could see Johnny Finger stand up, defeated and broken. As I focused on Johnny's battered figure, Pop's words rang in my head, "Life ain't cheap. A man has to pay a price to get what he wants."

Amen, Pop, amen.

15 The Classic Fighter

"He who fights with monsters might take care lest he thereby become a monster. And if you gaze for long into an abyss, the abyss gazes also into you."
— *Friedrich Nietzsche*

Like my stubbornness, I inherited another behavioral tendency that coursed through my family's veins and rose to the surface when ignited—a fighting spirit. Momma never backed down from a fight, and neither did Pop. In fact, Momma Nettie knew how to throw down without any hesitation, especially when it came to protecting her loved ones.

I was four years old. While playing with my action figures in the backyard, the next-door neighbor's Chihuahua dug a hole under the fence and made its way onto our property. Having a Napoleonic complex for biting anything or anyone in its path, the Chihuahua emitted a bark that sounded more like a car horn. Jumping out of my skin, I climbed onto the highest point that lent itself, a lawn chair. But this pathetic attempt for safety didn't discourage the furry bullet from charging toward me. I braced myself, yelling in terror, waiting for it to climb up and yank off a piece of my flesh.

In a flash, Momma Nettie darted from the house wielding a broom that knocked the tiny terror ten yards away. She continued her onslaught until the Chihuahua retreated under the fence.

Before she left the scene, Momma Nettie said to me, "All right, baby, now you can go back and play. Ain't no goddamn dog gonna bite you today."

A year later, Momma Nettie held me back from the second fight I witnessed up close and personal. It happened when our neighbor, Mrs. Marsha—who happened to be the owner of the

Chihuahua—came wobbling over to our house. She banged on the door, asking to see my mother. Obliging, Momma opened the screen door and confronted the two hundred pound Mrs. Marsha. According to our neighbor, her daughter and my brother got into an altercation a block away, where my brother pushed the eldest of Marsha's daughters off a curb after she scratched my brother's face. Over her yelling and the cigarette dangling from her mouth, Mrs. Marsha recounted the story and demanded that my brother come outside at once. Who knew what was behind Mrs. Marsha's semi-deranged state. Booze? High-stress? Anti-depressants? Whatever the reason, Mrs. Marsha was hysterical, and her intentions with my brother were not welcomed at our doorstep.

Responding in her calmest tone, Momma informed Mrs. Marsha that she wasn't going to see my brother under such circumstances. Before Momma could utter another syllable, our much larger neighbor took retribution to a different level by reeling back and slapping Momma in the face. Momma stumbled about, trying to gain her balance. Seeing the event unfold through the screen door, I called out to my mother from inside the house. Instantly, Momma Nettie took a hold of me, not allowing me to go near the fray.

Ever since she was a little girl, Momma was used to a sucker punch; she had been hit a lot harder by life, and by those who knocked her down verbally and physically for being a poor fatherless dago in her old neighborhood. One thing Momma learned in her younger days; if you get smacked, hit back harder.

Adhering to her school of hard knocks, Momma gained her composure, shifted her body, and came in with a roundhouse that clocked Mrs. Marsha, the cigarette, and her pride down onto the concrete; adding a peppery, "Now get the hell off my lawn, Marsha, before I really hurt you."

Crawling up on her knees and reaching for her bent cigarette, a more subdued Mrs. Marsha stood up and walked away with her tail between her legs, just like her Chihuahua.

According to Pop, he took the same approach when facing a confrontation. As glasses of Porto wine flushed through him on weekend nights, Pop reminisced about his youthful fights in the projects where names like "Spic Bastard" and "Brownie" would set off my fifteen-year old father like a bottle rocket. Like walking in hole-torn sneakers and working two jobs to feed his family, brawls on the corner were a daily routine during Pop's formative years. Later, he'd apply that same fighting spirit to something more constructive — The Marines.

So, when my family heard about "The Finger Incident," it was no surprise they took the news in stride. That evening at the dinner table, hours after my confrontation with Finger, I found myself staring at a pensive version of my father. He mulled over my story for a few moments, laced his fingers together, leaned over and asked, "Do you think you did the right thing, son?"

I nodded.

"Is that a yes sir, or a no sir?"

"Y-Y-Yes, sir."

"Good. You can sleep better tonight knowing you did a good thing." Pop then ordered me to go to bed.

Staring up at the rotating fan, guilt faded away as I lay in bed and replayed the events that had transpired hours prior. A thrill of liberation waked over me. I could return to school the following week, arch my back a bit more, and raise my chin a little higher instead of casting my eyes down, agonizing over Johnny's next ambush. I could face my fears, just like my parents and my great-grandmother did so many times before me. We were bent on fighting for something greater than ourselves. The satisfaction I found in those familial virtues helped me drift into a deep sleep.

Even though I begged Momma to keep "The Finger Incident" a secret from Momma Nettie, everything in me wanted to share my small victory with my great-grandmother of how I confronted my own Chihuahua. But I censored myself. I didn't want her to worry, or make her heart flutter erratically. Instead, I

resorted to sneaking into Momma Nettie's room and leaving a
plethora of uplifting sketches on her nightstand, as she wheezed
and moaned in her sleep.

Rumors spread like wildfire after our Spring Break, but this
time the buzz didn't involve my stuttering or how my parents
raised some monstrosity out of incest. On the contrary, word of
mouth circulated on how I beat the ever-loving crap out of
Johnny Finger and the Walter twins. I noticed a shift in the way
my peers looked at me. Respect permeated from their eyes.

There was one person who didn't fully embrace my Finger
confrontation with open arms. Learning of my brawl, Brother
Raphael approached me at lunch and asked me about the
dispute. Biting into my soggy sandwich, I retold the story. With
his hand on my head, Brother Raphael advised me, "Please come
to me next time it happens. Fights aren't always the answer. I
can help you, you know that?"

A part of me wanted to resent Brother's pacifist ideals. He
may not have known it, but there was a jungle out there and
because of my impediment, I was easy prey. I had to fight fire
with fire in order to survive. But even though Brother's ethos
intimidated me, I didn't have animosity towards him. He was a
man of God. He believed in turning the other cheek and
forgiving others seventy times seven. One day I would comply
with Brother's practices, but to buy into such divine notions
seemed weak and unbeneficial at the time. I didn't have the
luxury or the courage to follow his biblical rules.

Overlooking my tempestuous actions and holding true to his
promise, Brother Raphael did help me in his own way by skipping
over me during the reading aloud assignments. Like Ms. Marquez,
my fifth-grade teacher randomly selected boys in class instead of
going row by row. This kept Brother Raphael's favoritism towards
me as discreet as possible, and simmered any future conflicts that
may have arisen between the other students and me.

Another way Brother cared for me was by offering me his
devoted time and his wealth of knowledge. Because of his

sapient insight, Brother Raphael was fully aware of my fixation with the books he assigned to us. Maybe Brother overheard me reading alone in class during lunch, or caught glimpses of me by the school pond's embankment as I whispered written words to myself. In those times of solace, I savored in my diction of words and the smoothness that emanated from my voice. When I knew no condemning ears were present, I attained elocution. My insecurities didn't clutter my mind, and I gave myself the right to move seamlessly among the written word. But what are words when you can't share them with others?

It wasn't long after that my mentor joined me during my reading time, where we extracted and discussed in-depth themes from the assigned classics. Carrying over to my second year at the academy, our time together evolved into a much-anticipated part of my day. I recall one random afternoon where I explained my viewpoint on a particular mythological story, "N-N-Narcis-s-sus w-was t-t-too much int-t-to um, um, himself."

"Yes, lad. You are correct." Brother agreed. "That's why he drowned. Sometimes when we become self-centered, we drown in ourselves. But God did not intend us to be that way. He made us to help others."

Brother had a talent for turning any topic into something biblical, and he made it a point to live by those lessons. Like a message on a mound, his enlightenment inspired me to further excavate the meaning behind literature, and apply those lessons to my life. My mind expanded, and my imagination skyrocketed as I read the books not only assigned to me, but the books that my older brother left around after starting high school. My literary film flickered and illuminated in my mind as I created the visuals from the words that splashed across the pages.

On some occasions, Brother asked me to read dialogue from the plays we were studying, with a little help from my acquired accents, of course—just the two of us and a magnolia tree flourishing above us, while the ruckus of boys playing soccer echoed in the distance. From *Oedipus Rex* to *Antigone*, we covered a gambit of plays that pushed the limits of my ten-year old mind and the quality of my voice. Most of the time I couldn't comprehend exactly what I was reading, but I loved the poetic, rhythmic, and often challenging words on my lips.

Not all of my time at the Academy entailed understanding, acceptance, and everyone singing "Kumbaya." During the second and third week of sixth-grade, Finger taunted me again, hungering for a rematch, even after a year had passed. Whatever the reason for his rematch, his reputation was marred and he demanded retribution. When Finger did finally corner me, he found me in an unprepared situation.

If I wasn't with Brother Raphael under the magnolia tree during lunch, anyone could locate me in the sixth-grade homeroom pronouncing words from a book while chomping away at my peanut butter and jelly sandwich. On a particular afternoon, the crashing of two desks behind me interrupted my serenity. "You talking to yourself, stutterbird?!"

Without even thinking, I turned to confront Johnny Finger. But there wasn't enough time to dodge his fist from descending upon my face. The punch twirled me around, while the ache in my cheek throbbed. *Did my face just fall off?* I pondered as the dizziness momentarily set in. It was the first time someone had hit me in the face.

Suddenly, the wooziness faded and the rage surged. As red hazed my vision, I blocked out Brother's lessons on forgiveness. Consumed with vengeance, I clipped Finger in the stomach with an uppercut, causing his body to career into the desks. By this time, faces filled the French door windows to witness the rematch between Finger and The Hulk.

Grabbing Finger by the shirt, I spun him around and threw him into the wooden desks. I heard the "oohs" echo from behind the window. An excitement filled me, and I relished in the attention. If I was going to have a reputation, I'd rather it be one of a bruiser than of a stutterer who pissed in his pants.

Finger asked me to stop, but sympathy wasn't invited to this pow-wow. I clenched my fingers around Johnny's greasy hair and slammed his cranium onto the desk. Before I inflicted any more injury upon Finger, someone had already pulled me off of my nemesis. "Stop it! Now!"

Snapping out of my frenzy, I found a mortified Brother Andrews — one of our Social Science teachers — looking down at me. Yanking me by the arm and down the corridor, Andrews told me that he had no other choice but to report the incident.

We were headed to the principal's office.

This time Momma was called in. Sitting outside of the principal's office, I reverted back to years prior when I sat in waiting rooms while Momma and pathologist were on the other side of the door, discussing my future. But unlike those days, I didn't feel shame about my voice as I paced around the principal's waiting room. Instead, I clung onto a different disappointment. My family's name had been tarnished, and this time it wasn't of my brother's doing.

Before I had a chance to wallow in regret, I heard Momma's voice escalate from behind the principal's door, similar to when she and Pop argued, or when she raised her voice when my brother and I rambunctiously ran around the house. Minutes later, Momma rushed out of the office, reached for my hand and led me to the car. By the aggravation on her face I could tell the meeting didn't go well.

Unlike my first main event, my parents had a different response to my second round with Johnny Finger. Pop may have understood my frustrations, but he scolded me nevertheless, telling me I had to control my temper. Momma gave me the same speech, even though she told our principal that just because Johnny Sr. had been a main contributor to the school, it didn't give his son the right to pick on whomever he pleased. But the principal ignored Momma's logic and stated that the next time I participated in any fight, I would be suspended for a week. I guess the principal's back pocket ran deeper than his moral convictions.

I had no more lifelines, no more "get out of jail free" cards. What happened to the good boy? I'll tell you what happened to him, his back was against the wall, and he had no more room for errors. The Incredible Hulk had been evicted, never to return again. I had no other choice but to control the rage, even when instigated. But how could I crush the inherited fighting spirit that coursed through me? How could I demand respect from bullies without my fists, and with only stuttering words at my disposal?

It would take a subtle intervention from my white-bearded mentor to soothe my anger. Soon, Brother Raphael would put my fighting spirit to better use by unlocking a new door to my future, and honing my vigor and angst toward a more productive goal. It seemed as if I had one more lifeline left after all.

16 Thank You, Sandy Duncan

"Man may have discovered fire, but women discovered how to play with it."
— *Candace Bushnell*, Sex & The City

I can't do this.

This was the delusional thought that plagued me as I stood backstage, waiting for my cue. With familiar nerves cramping my stomach, I weighed my options—running out of the gymnasium-turned-theater and hiding under the magnolia tree, or taking a bus and going home. My choices to escape were endless and somewhat tempting, yet I couldn't ignore the reality hanging in the air. In a few minutes, I had to say the lines, and this time I didn't have Pauley rescuing me from my responsibilities. Brother Raphael depended on me to get on stage and perform to the best of my abilities. I owed him that much. Hell, I owed it to myself.

I didn't end up in this precarious situation by my own doing; it took the subtle persuasion of my prep-school mentor to coerce me. Entering my last semester of sixth grade at Christian Brothers Academy, Brother Raphael and I continued our literary summits, even though I no longer had Brother as a teacher in any of my sixth grade classes. During one encounter in the spring of '85, Brother surprised me with a challenging opportunity.

All around me, books slapped shut and desks scraped against the tiled floor as students pushed from their seats. Book bags swung over shoulders and students rushed out of the classroom in a matter of seconds, making their way to lunch. I, on the other hand, had other priorities. Remaining in my seat, I ignored the rumbling in my stomach as I devoured the words of a mythological story that had me in its grasp.

Greeting students who darted past him, Brother Raphael entered the classroom and made his way toward me. Usually he and I met a half hour into the lunch period, so his abrupt and early arrival was most unexpected.

"Good one, huh?" Brother asked me, referring to the Perseus and Pegasus story that lay open in front of me. A few niceties were exchanged between us before Brother Raphael leaned in, and placed a New Testament reference book as well as a folded piece of paper on top of my desk. "The play is coming up next month, and since I'm directing it this year, I would be honored for you to play a pivotal role."

The play Brother referred to was a staged version of various biblical stories from the New Testament, where students from fifth to seventh grade sported robes and sashes, and portrayed the likes of Christ, Peter, and Mary. To be in such a production was a high honor in the school, yet dread was all I tasted in Brother's offer.

Opening the creased paper, Brother showed me my lines. I'm sure he saw fear glazing over my eyes and instant tension in my body. "I know about your dilemma, but I am certain you can play this role," Brother affirmed. "You've used those voices so many times with me, and you understand this type of material. I know you can do this, lad."

Brother gently placed his hand on my shoulder, as if he offered me some sort of blessing. On the top of the page, it read: Queen Herodias: "Give me his head on a platter. I want John the Baptist's head! You owe me that much, my king."

That was all, three sentences. Yet the bad no-no's popped out at me…G, P, I, J, B, K. The dialogue looked like a long stretch of highway, impossible words to conquer. No way could I say those letters in front of an audience with my normal voice. Even if I used an accent, what would happen then? Never before had I acted out such lines in front of strangers, or worse, in front of the whole student body. Added to the mix was the uncertainty that came when portraying a queen. I repeatedly asked myself how could I play a woman? I'd probably urinate on myself again, or worse, vomit in the midst of two hundred students.

As I sank in my desk and reviewed my current state of affairs, Brother never took his eyes off of me, "You have passion, my dear boy. Let's apply it to more constructive things, yes?"

Taking Brother's Raphael's advice to heart, I spent the following days methodically reading excerpts from the biblical reference book. Pages upon pages described the history of Queen Herodias — how she loathed John the Baptist, who denounced her love affair with King Herod, Herodias' brother-in-law. The theme reminded me of *Richard III*, and the Greek tragedies I read and discussed in-length with Brother. I loved the twisted emotions of the characters, the drama, the incest, and the scandal. The tension between Herodias and John the Baptist was profound, and the conflict fed my appetite for complex storytelling. The more I invested in the characters, the less I stressed over the stuttering and the opinions of others, especially from Johnny Finger.

Sketches upon sketches gushed out of me as I returned to my dependable medium. Envisioning Queen Herodias and her postures, I drew her physical mannerisms in my sketchbook. Proud of my creations, I showed my renderings to Brother while I discussed Herodias' vengeful traits and how her vanity led to her demise. My mentor listened to my ongoing chatter with a prideful smile and an amused chuckle.

A week before opening night, the excitement diminished and another form of resistance arose. How could I, an eleven-year-old boy, embody the elegance of a woman on stage? Could I pull it off or was I way over my head? Even if I could, I panicked at the thought of acting out feminine gestures in an all-boys school. For so long, I tried to earn a reputation of being strong and resilient against bullies, and now I was giving them fodder to use against me. "The stutterer who likes to wear dresses." I could hear it now. I was committing hara-kiri!

Tossing and turning in my bed, a memory suddenly roused me from my semi-slumber, a memory that I should've recalled but didn't until the witching hour. It was the first professional play I had ever attended. Seeing her in green tights, short blonde hair, and pixie dust,

I instantly fell in love with the woman who played the boy from Neverland. Sandy Duncan flew above my six-year old head, sprinkling dreams and wonderment down onto the audience. My senses soared and the audience cheered as the actress embodied the playfulness of a boy, gliding with happy thoughts and glowing with not a care in the world. The packed auditorium stood, applauded, and reached out to her as she sang, "I'm Flying." Sandy Duncan personified perfection because of her commitment to the role.

If a then twenty-something year old actress could personify Peter Pan on a national tour of the same name, why couldn't I do the opposite—a boy portraying a queen in a biblical play? Sure, the jeers and insults would follow, but if I wanted to take the next step into fluency, I had to commit to the duty at hand. I was determined to roll the dice and see where my fate landed.

Minutes before my entrance on stage, I finally gathered up my courage and put the situation into its proper perspective. I stared at my reflection in the long mirror that was nailed to the gymnasium wall. I was adorned with pieces of silk that draped down to my ankles, a gold band that wrapped around my forehead, and a tight white shirt around my body.

I arched my back and raised my chin. Like a queen, my posture embodied regality. I whispered my three lines over and over. My voice may have had a higher pitch, but it carried girth. I looked and sounded like a woman who wanted a prophet's head on a platter. When no one was around, I sounded clear, just like all those other times I read alone. But in front of the packed gymnasium, a different outcome awaited me, I was sure of it. *If only I could block them out, and make them disappear until I said my last line*, I wondered as I heard my cue filter from the stage.

With commitment in my body, and persistency on my mind, I parted the curtains and entered the stage. Win or lose, I was going to give it my all. As the fervor outweighed the fear, I leapt into the void; the artist's journey had begun.

As my scene transpired on stage, I was somewhere else. It all occurred in the blink of an eye. I operated on something instinctual, forgetting what happened the previous second. What I do remember is diverting my attention away from the audience and blocking out the sea of faces. I didn't want to make eye contact with any of them, especially Momma, who I knew was out there among the viewers. If I did look out, the lunch I'd eaten an hour ago would most assuredly make a visit on stage, so I focused on my dialect and the other student playing King Herod. Placing my voice in a different register with an English flare to it, I tried to leap over my bad no-no's. Perfect fluency didn't stream from my mouth in those three lines, and of course, buffers like "um's" and "you see's" projected out, but I did it. It wasn't perfect, but dammit it, I did it.

It would take lowering my adrenaline and calming my shivering nerves to truly assess my achievement. Once off stage, I replayed the performance in my mind. I had said rehearsed lines in front of an audience without cowering away and without the violent convulsions that usually came with the stuttering. My love for storytelling ascended to new heights, beyond my "Movie Players" group, and beyond my wildest expectations.

Thank you, Sandy Duncan.

Outside in the school's courtyard, kids and parents embraced one another. The scent of coffee and pastries filled the air, reminding me of Momma Nettie and her infamous chicory coffee. I couldn't wait to see her and share my triumphant day with her. Darting toward my elated mother, I wrapped my arms around her waist as she congratulated me.

Looking over to the side, I saw Brother Raphael from across the courtyard. I locked eyes with him as he extended his signature thumbs toward me. He never said it, but I knew he was thinking, "You did it, lad."

The silent cheer we exchanged from across the courtyard would be one of the last times I'd see my scholarly mentor. As seventh grade approached, Brother Raphael and I would end our literary summits. I guess he realized I had learned all I could from him. Soon—like many of the Brothers at Christian Brothers—Raphael would slip into obscurity, passing into the solitude of a world that would change and have no place for a old-fashioned literary gentleman. I still imagine Raphael's last days, walking the green gardens of the retirement home, pondering Ulysses' quest for glory, articulating the words of Homer, and the birds singing in unison to Raphael's delicious diction. I think of such timeless, immortal things with a bittersweet sentiment. Even years later, I pause and meditate on my angelic, baldheaded mentor who opened the flood gates to my miraculous discovery, who unsealed a world of literature to my limited mind, and who gave me the greatest gift any human could give another human, time — committed, selfless time.

As I acknowledged Brother Raphael, Momma turned and saw the beaming reaction from my mentor. Momma returned a wave as well.

"Let's go say hi," said Momma.

Something in me didn't want to, though. For me, his subtle smile and his thumbs up was enough. It was his delicate and clever way of not saying too much, but saying everything at the same time. Sometimes the best words are left unsaid.

"N-N-No, I want t-t-to go t-t-tell M-Momma N-Nettie about wh-what happened."

Momma's face went rigid. Her pursed lips and squinty eyes was a reaction I knew all too well. Kneeling next to me, Momma told me that Momma Nettie had to return to the hospital. She hadn't told me earlier because she didn't want to upset me before my big performance. Momma paused for moment, and then said, "But let's tell her when she gets home, okay?"

"Wh-Wh-en will that be?"

17 Behind the Green Curtain

"Our dead are never dead to us, until we have forgotten them."
— *George Eliot*

Momma Nettie died on a fall morning, a few months after my portrayal of Herodias. During those months, her body rapidly depleted. Some days she lay up in her bedroom, while other nights she remained comatose in a hospital room. I waited for the right time to tell her about my accomplishments and to resume our weekend TV watching. I never got the chance to do either.

To keep me calm, my parents downplayed Momma Nettie's condition, never allowing me to go visit her in the hospital or disturb her in her room. All that time I thought Momma Nettie's cancer was in remission, yet I never knew the severity of her illness until the night my parents told me she had peacefully passed away. I sat speechless. I didn't know what to say or how to convey the betrayal I felt in my heart.

For so long my family coddled me and continued to keep valuable information away from me. Was I that fragile? Was I that incompetent to deal with Momma Nettie's illness? Did the stuttering make me into a whimpering, faint-hearted boy that had to be handled with surgical gloves?

They didn't tell me about the blackness taking over Nettie's lungs, liver, and esophagus. All those nights of countless drinks and cigarettes took their toll on my great-grandmother. I witnessed her incessant intake firsthand, but at that age I didn't know the meaning of self-abuse, especially living in New Orleans where relentless drinking and smoking were customary activities. Momma Nettie's habits went under the radar, hidden behind days filled with raising two boys and weekly bingo games, while her nights consisted of regret and heartbreak. Locking herself in her room, she desperately muffled those nighttime demons that whispered to her during her binges, reminding her of an ex-husband whom she still loved, and of the dreams she never achieved. During our sleepovers, I remember overhearing her faint mumbles as I went in and out of sleep.

My initial feeling of betrayal simmered as her funeral approached, and slowly another emotion revealed its rancid face: I began to blame myself for her death.

Even as I was about to turn twelve, I couldn't grasp the meaning behind my ludicrous feelings. Who could at such an age? Severe guilt was just a normal response that I had grown accustomed to whenever something went awry. My continual guilt stemmed from how I viewed myself as a problem—a delinquent in a serene suburb.

Reflecting back thirty years later, I can finally articulate what I thought during that time of grief. Because I wasn't a good boy, I assumed Momma Nettie left us in response to my disobedience. As much as I tried to keep my secrets from her, she was—in my mind--an omnipresent being, always aware of my erratic behaviors. The list of my wrongdoings raced through my conscience for weeks—violently beating Finger twice, yelling at Momma and Pop when the stuttering was too much to bear, lashing out at my brother when he took his books back, sipping on church wine before I dressed in my altar boy robe, allowing my impediment to get the best of me, and never spending more time with Momma Nettie during her last days. To me, her death symbolized my wrongdoings. If only she felt the grasp of my hand or the warmth of my voice during her battle with cancer, maybe she would've fought earnestly to live. If only I was a good boy.

Little did I know, Momma Nettie's choices led to her demise. Drinking and smoking were part of her coping. Yet to blame such a divine person like Momma Nettie as being flawed was blasphemy in my limited scope. It was easier to give into my co-dependency and lay the liability on me. I had become an expert in that realm.

The day came to lay her to rest. The indoor mausoleum smelled like wilting flowers. The tang stung my nostrils as I squeezed my nose shut, blocking out the annoying scent. We followed her casket while they wheeled it to her tomb. A long line of tombs surrounded us, but I couldn't look at them. Any minute now, Momma Nettie would join them—the marble slab, the spider webs, and the darkness.

The coffin stopped in front of a small green curtain. The emerald cloth hid the horizontal abyss where her silver casket would rest. I wanted to rip the curtain open, climb in there and make sure this was all a joke. The Wizard of Oz must be behind the curtain, planning this, lying to us, and making us think this was our reality. Maybe if I clicked my heels three times, Momma Nettie would be sitting home, waiting for me to eat her red beans and rice while she sipped on scotch.

Locking the wheels, the pallbearers picked up the coffin. My brother broke down; he was the first one to lose it. *Why was he crying?* I wondered. My brother had his friends, his theater group, and his girlfriend, while my life rolled by me in a tin box, and slid into a crypt, behind the green curtain.

The emotional weight from Momma Nettie's death kept me in a depressed solitude, not only from the guilt, but because my stuttering, once again, took a turn for the worse. Both guilt and stuttering worked hand-in-hand with one another, one feeding the other until they led to their ultimate goal—a shameful silence. Just when I thought I had conquered my impediment during my biblical performance, I teetered back to my old ways. The bad no-no's re-emerged, and they unrelentingly stumped me for months to come. In the process, I found a new masochistic habit to cope with my stuttering as I turned twelve.

Like revving up a lawnmower by tugging on a pull chord, I yanked on my hair, trying to pull the word out of me when I hit a troubled spot. When this form of self-abuse occurred, Momma or Pop would leap toward me, stopping me from my fits. The wrenching of the hair and my persistent yelling continued for almost a year. Sooner or later, Momma had to force her hand into the matter.

Momma knew I had to vent out in a more constructive way, yet her patience was wearing thin. She was grieving as well, and my outbursts didn't help. At her wits end, Momma told me that since the stammering had gotten worse, and since I was going to leave Christian Brothers that following spring in '86, maybe speaking with a professional would be a better option. The thought of visiting a psychiatrist forced my sensibilities to go berserk. Seeing a shrink meant I had hit a disastrous point in the eyes of my family. Only crazy or troubled people talked to psychiatrists, and what usually followed were a barrage of other charming factors—drugs, institutions, shock treatment, and padded walls. Perhaps I'd watched *One Flew Over the Cookoo's Nest* one too many times on late night television.

After much consideration, I vehemently said no. The thought of a doctor prodding and asking preposterous questions didn't stick well with my childlike impatience. I had been to that circus several times before, especially with pathologists and other specialists as the ringleaders. I knew my present situation was different, and I needed a more creative outlet to release the tension; I needed to get lost in the stories that helped me forget my reality. But where could I find such opportunities? There was no Pauley, and no Brother Raphael offering me a role of a lifetime. Thus, loneliness had shoved itself upon me even more.

When I expressed my reservations about not seeing a psychiatrist, Momma didn't press the point any further. I may have stuttered, but when I felt something deeply, anyone could detect my meaning by the conviction in my eyes; at least that part of my communication had clarity.

Since I couldn't talk to anyone about my grief, I drastically closed myself off. In my solitude, I fervently sketched pictures of

Momma Nettie. For months, I'd draw images of her from older sepia toned snapshots when Nettie posed with Santa Claus, or ones of Momma Nettie holding Momma when she was a toddler. Sketching her lessened the guilt. My heartache told me that if her features stayed on my pages, then maybe she would live forever.

At night when I wrestled with heavy thoughts, I began to converse with my immortal sketches of Momma Nettie stashed under my bed. Before drifting to a sleep, I'd slide the sketches out and speak freely and stutter-free to them. If someone happened to spy on me or barge into my room, they would've witnessed a crazy sight—a kid having a conversation with drawn pictures as tears and laughs streamed out of him. Insane or not, I found something cathartic and comforting in the nighttime ritual. Sometimes I heard Momma Nettie among the chirping crickets and the wind brushing against my window, telling me that she was happy, and that all was forgiven. I don't know what comforted me more, connecting with my dear great-grandmother, or hearing my words come out with fluency.

The urge to hurt myself gradually diminished, and soon, I put an end to my hair pulling. Perhaps speaking to my sketches did have a positive influence after all, but it didn't shrink the loneliness that still clung to me. Forcing a smile when I desperately wanted to connect with the living became a normal inner desperation. To hide this feeling of disconnection, I played the part of the good boy once again—any part was better than going to a specialist or being a distressed child in the eyes of my grieving parents.

Since Christian Brothers and other prep schools in the New Orleans area ended at seventh grade, selected private high schools offered eighth grade classes for students. So ready or not, as the end of my stay with Christian Brothers neared, a new drastic adjustment blasted its way into my life, the world of high school—full of all its awkwardness and discomfort. But instead of starting my new environment with enthusiasm, I prepared for the inevitable jeers and slanders. In a Pavlovian way, my past history conditioned me to expect the insults that would most assuredly come my way.

Just eight blocks from where we lived, Archbishop Rummel High School — a Catholic high school — was the staple for strict education in our neighborhood. During those first days as I made my way down the hallways, I felt like a moving target to the many faces that passed by me. In retaliation, I didn't want to know them, either. For all I knew, one of them could've been the next Finger lurking about.

As a form of self-preservation, I stayed in my seat, listened to the lessons, ate lunch alone, and went about my day while shutting myself off from everyone around me. And since my birthday landed in November, most of my classmates had almost a year on me. They were growing in spurts and hitting puberty way before me. My still chubby, short stature contrasted with everyone around me. Thus, my only goal was to ebb and flow out of the all-boy high school with as little attention drawn to my appearance and my stuttering as possible.

I missed Brother Raphael more than ever.

18 To Sing the Impossible Song

"I only sing in the shower. I would join a choir, but I don't think my bathtub can hold that many people."
— Jarod Kintz

Ignoring my stammering protests, Momma tried to pull me out of my isolated cave by forcing me into a more social situation, which sounded as appealing as getting a tetanus shot. According to Momma, extra-curricular activities would help strengthen my self-esteem and build stronger friendships along the way. As she so eloquently explained, "If you're not going to see a psychiatrist, then you're sure as hell gonna have to make friends. But you're not gonna to spend your days locked away in your room."

Hence, in the fall of 1986 as I approached my thirteenth birthday, Momma wanted me to join the Catholic Youth Organization (CYO), a local group that not only served those in need, but also brought youths together in a secured atmosphere, like supervised dances and other social activities. At first, I had no intentions of volunteering or wasting my time watching adolescents dance their Saturday nights away. But after some consideration, I reluctantly went along with Momma's not-so-subtle suggestion and became a member of St. Benilde's CYO chapter. Besides feeding the homeless and monitoring bingo nights for the elderly, my reasons for joining the CYO were of a selfish nature—to keep Momma satisfied and calm, while biding some time until my family stopped worrying about my inability to fit in.

CYO meetings took place every Sunday night after the youth mass, a CYO sponsored service where the choir performed songs from *Godspell*, *Jesus Christ Superstar*, and other religious musicals. Being a devout Vatican One follower—including never touching the

Eucharist with her hands, always genuflecting when the tabernacle opened, and believing that shaking hands during "The Peace Be With You" portion of the mass paralleled "drunkards high-fiving each other at a bar"—Momma thought the rock n' roll choir was too secular for a Catholic mass. I, on the other hand, took great delight in the choir's panache and the familiar songs they brought to the drab service.

Before my brother moved to New York for college, musical recordings—ranging from *Into The Woods* to *Hello Dolly*—were a part of my everyday home life. Disregarding others in the house, my brother would blare his vinyl Broadway records while holding the whole household hostage to his music selections. In time, I became an accidental aficionado to almost every musical written. So it was no surprise that during the religious services, I sang with heartfelt pleasure, knowing the lyrics by heart, with sureness and without stuttering. Pointing my attention to the choir loft—which was located just to the side of the altar—I belted out words that easily streamed from my mouth. Hambuga and her lyrical influence affectionately passed through my thoughts.

At the end of the service, as most of the youthful congregation rushed out to attend the CYO meeting, I'd linger, singing and clapping the last hymn. Watching the choir break down microphones, drums, and amplifiers, I shook with anticipation. So badly I wanted to approach one of the members of the choir and ask them if I could join their company of singers and musicians. But would they take me seriously if I stammered and peddled my way through the question? They would most assuredly judge me by how I spoke and not by how I sang. With my trepidation ultimately being the victor, I decided the pew would be my sanctuary for the time being.

During those first CYO meetings, I stayed hush-hush and inattentive, like a parolee passing his hours of community service. While I hid in the back row, I studied the members around me, consisting mostly of my former classmates from St. Benilde. Puberty changed many of their features; some of the girls looked like models, while some of the boys had slight peach fuzz gracing their upper lips and a deeper cadence to their voices. To them, I was probably a stranger as well, but instead of growing tall, I was filling out horizontally. Part of me hoped they wouldn't recognize me. The last time they laid eyes on me I was a stammering buffoon who played with toys and hung around oddballs.

During one unforgettable meeting as I leaned back on my chair and balanced my seat on its two back legs, I saw a large figure out of the corner of my eye rush toward me. Taking me by surprise, I almost fell off my chair when his loud voice shook me out of my isolation.

"Well, look what the cat dragged in," said the familiar voice.

Regaining my balance on the chair, I looked up. I recognized the chubby cheeks, the doggie eyes, and the gangly arms. There, lingering above me was a taller and more mature-looking Pauley. A jolt of excitement blasted through me as I jumped up and embraced him. Pauley was a sight for sore eyes, and assessing how he hugged me and cackled out his signature laugh, I could tell my childhood friend was thrilled to see me as well.

In the confines of the back row, we caught up on the past three years. Pauley's stories contained the trials he endured during and after St. Benilde — being picked on for his weight, his Mom passing away, and how he was learning to adjust to his new high school. My tales consisted of similar themes as we bonded through our war stories. Our long-lost camaraderie warmed over me and fed my hunger for acceptance.

My weekends found new adventures with my old, yet trusty partner in crime. Besides volunteering our time with the CYO's outreach programs — which we found more gratifying than we had previously expected — Pauley and I resumed our movie watching, either at the theaters or on our new VHS machines. Besides films, our interests in the arts grew deeper as we whisked into 1987. Sometimes we boomed out Billy Joel,

Bruce Springsteen, and Chicago through the record player, sipping on their poetic lyrics about love and lost. Occasionally, Pauley sang fervently with the music and I joined in as well with a splash of harmony.

One afternoon, as Pauley and I blasted Peter Cetera's tenor voice through my stereo, and we hit the high notes in unison, an idea popped into my head: What if we joined the choir together? But in mere seconds I wiped the preposterous idea from my thoughts. How would a stuttering buffoon and a clumsy, overweight kid live up to the choir's reputation? People listened to the choir every Sunday. People clapped and sang with them. People never gave Pauley or me a second glance.

During one of our visits to the mall, Pauley and I sucked down Orange Julius drinks as we popped coins into arcade games. Making our pixelated figures zigzag about the screen, we tugged on the machine's joysticks. Suddenly, out of nowhere, Pauley came up with a poignant plan. "You wanna join the choir on Sunday nights with me?"

His question slapped me in the face. "A-A-Are you s-s-serious?" I asked while my hand froze on the joystick.

Pauley was as serious as a heart attack. To prove his conviction, he told me that he knew the choir director—some young hipster who lent his musical talents to the Sunday night services. To this day I don't remember the connection between Pauley and the choir director; all I do recall is that Pauley stayed true to his word by asking the director if we could join.

A few days later, nerves and anticipation rocked through my body as Pauley told me the good news—we were official members of the choir. Sooner than expected, Pauley and I found ourselves singing in the back of the choir loft. I didn't care if I was in the very front or as far away as Istanbul. I wasn't asking to be in the limelight. To be in that choir loft was just as rewarding as being on a Broadway stage. In my tiny, flimsy world, I had made the big time.

Unlike Pauley, who peered down at the sheet music as he followed along note by note, I had a different approach to my singing. Closing my eyes and singing from memory, I savored every note vibrating in my throat. The same electrical feeling I had on the stage at Christian Brothers was coursing through me once again. For the first time in years, I didn't feel like a boy who struggled with his words. In the eyes of the congregation, I was a normal kid who sang with ease. Concealing my dysfunction behind the music, I loved the intoxication that came with performing and I didn't want it to end. After every Sunday mass, I couldn't wait for my next week's injection of bliss.

Along with my weekly choir time, I learned to cope with the stress that came with high school as well as my home life. I finally had an artistic outlet to release my anxieties and worries. As I grew more confident with my singing and less agitated with my impediment, I found myself feeling the music in a more profound way during those Sunday night services. The words resonated with me on a higher level, and my emotional connection was evident in my dramatic interpretation; my loud clapping and gestures reflected something out of a musical production.

Maybe that was why the most beautiful girl I had ever laid eyes on took notice of me as she sat in the third row of the congregation. At first I thought she was staring at someone else, but as soon as I locked eyes with her, she imprisoned me. On that particular Sunday night where dreams cluttered reality, I had my first nibble at romance, and my first admittance into that majestic, yet petrifying realm called infatuation.

19 I'm Not Tom Cruise

"Nothing ends nicely, that's why it ends."
—*Tom Cruise*

Married since 1966, Momma and Pop were never the overtly romantic types. They exchanged kisses, and embraced each other when the moment called for it, but the cuddling and the wooing were never practiced out in the open. The closest to romantic interludes came when I witnessed my parents slow dance at their wedding anniversary party, and when they locked lips as they rung in the New Year. Whenever we watched TV as a family, they never held hands or stroked each other's hair. Instead, they lounged on opposite sides of the living room, two separate points of disinterest. Niceties said in a humdrum tone like, "I love you" before bed, and "Dinner was great, hun," were thrown into the mix, but romance— passionate, pursued affection—hardly existed between Pop and Momma. They acted more like roommates than as husband and wife.

So asking my parents about girls and crushes seemed like a taboo matter to discuss. I assumed they wouldn't comprehend such fanciful notions since they never practiced it. Besides, their response would probably be one of coddling, warning me about the complexities and stings that love had to offer. In their opinion—or so I assumed—the world never openly embraced a kid with a speech impediment. To them I was a fragile case that would most assuredly get used, taken advantage of, and brushed aside by a pretty face.

After seeing the luminous brunette at church, an obsession grew, and my lovely agony couldn't be ignored. The songs I sang either at church or with Pauley in the confines of my room were dedicated to the nameless brunette. My sketches of mountain landscapes and angelic creatures flying on clouds were not for me anymore, they were for the girl I made eye contact with on Sunday nights.

The more I thought of her, the more I fixated on movies that painted love affairs with thrilling and vivid strokes. In time, films like *The Karate Kid* and *Top Gun* became my great educator when dealing with the matter of the heart. No more did I focus on the car explosions and knife wielding fight scenes. My attention turned to themes where a man fought for the woman, fought for her integrity, and earned her hand. In the end, the guy always ended up with the girl. The aches and passions between the cinematic men and women conjured up a poetic spirit within me. A confidence emerged, more adventurous than anything I could've imagined. Ignoring my limited voice and the embarrassment that came with my dysfunction, I was determined to express my feelings and live a romantic life.

On a spring evening in '87 as the Huey Lewis tune pulsated through the speakers and a disco ball swirled above Pauley and me, I was ready to make a bold move. From across the rec center, she looked like a blurred vision, even though I knew her features by heart. Ever since I first laid eyes on her at church, she plagued my thoughts, and immediately I had to know the name of my infatuation.

Later I would discover her name—Mary.

The upbeat Huey Lewis song ended, and without warning, a ballad followed. I knew the ballad all too well; it was one of the songs Pauley and I played over and over until we wore out the record, "Take My Breath Away." The familiarity with the song brought a smile to my face; it was from *Top Gun*.

In an instant, the dance floor cleared. When a slow song played at the CYO dances, an abrupt exodus from the dance area occurred. No one dared take the initiative to be the first one to slow dance. But I didn't care. The mission outweighed the opinions of others. As people shoved pass me, I made my way toward her. I was going to ask Mary to dance.

My chest heaved in and out, trying to sustain some constant airflow. For a moment, I closed my eyes and allowed the music to stimulate my imagination—my only salvation. Instantly, I was transported to another time and another movie. I wore a bomber jacket, sunglasses, and sported a perfectly trimmed body. Resembling Tom Cruise, I could see Mary waiting for me on the side of a street as the wind blew through her hair and the sunset rays danced on her cheeks.

The picture became so crystal clear in my head:

Fade in: Mary Anne jumps on Scott's black and gold bicycle as she holds onto Scott. Scott peddles into the sunset. The beauty kisses Scott on the back of the neck. They live happily ever after. Fade out...

Some had religion, while others had sports to inspire them to greater heights. I had movies.

I neared her and the name blurted out of me, "M-M-M-Mary!"

As she turned and faced me, the fragrance of her hair penetrated my nose. It intoxicated me, and with an inquisitive look to her face, she leaned into me. "What did you say, Scotty? I couldn't hear you over the music."

She called me Scotty, like a pet name, like we had known each other for years. The question raced through my mind: *Do you want to dance?* But like many times before, a bad no-no popped up like a spurt from a geyser. D's...those damn D's. Suddenly, my tongue stiffened, my throat clenched up, and my lips couldn't move. Instinctively, the replacements rallied together, and my mouth followed suit, "G-Go on floor. You and m-m-me?"

I sounded like Yoda by how I mismatched words around, but at least I got the point across. By Mary's narrow eyes, I couldn't tell if she was thrown off by my query, or flattered that I asked her to dance. To clarify my point, I extended my hand out, gesturing to the dance floor.

Mary's eyes widened. "You want me to dance with you?" she asked.

I nodded. Sliding her hand into mine, Mary gently led me to the dance floor, acting as if it was her idea all along. Like touching an electrical wire, a surge ran through me when she touched my hand. The next two minutes were blurred as my head became murky, smothered in a cloud of disbelief. Dancing with a girl was one thing, but having a girl—*the* girl—wrap her arms around my shoulders as we glided to the music was something out of the movies. Normal guys danced with pretty girls, not stuttering overweight kids. There was hope after all for my freakish voice and my extreme sensibilities, as I held the pinnacle of my dreams in my arms.

After the song ended, Mary thanked me and crossed into the blinding glare of the lights that reflected off the dance floor. A few seconds later, Pauley elbowed me from behind, "How was it?"

"M-M-Magical."

That night, Pauley slept over. No more were our midnight conversations consumed with Star Wars trivia or the weekend's blockbuster. Locking ourselves in my room, we spoke about our muses—his was a girl who lived just around the corner from my house, mine lived six blocks away. So badly we wanted to knock on their windows and express our undying love to them. Instead, over and over again, we replayed *The Karate Kid*, hoping that our existence could reflect Ralph Machio's roller coaster life. Upon watching the movie for the umpteenth time, I devised a plan—a tricky, risky strategy that would push me to a new level. When it came to the matters of the heart, there was no room for boundaries or reality, especially for a stutterer who was in love with love.

I'll admit it, at thirteen, I didn't know anything about being in love, yet something inside of me burst to life when my eyes set on Mary. I longed to harness that feeling, bottle it up, and drink it forever. Since Momma Nettie's death, I needed a woman to believe in me again, to give me a purpose to do my best, and to inspire me to express my feelings, forgoing any hesitation that came with my impediment. Every guy needed his leading lady, and on a muggy, bright summer morning, my bike and my determination charged forward to win the heart of a leading lady.

My hands gripped the handlebars of my bicycle as I turned the corner. I screeched to a halt in front of her house, hopped off the bike and pressed down on the kickstand. Lugging my backpack, I crossed to the door, and knocked. Mary's Mom answered. In my stuttering fashion, I asked if Mary could come to the door. Impatiently waiting, I pulled the boom box from out of my backpack and placed a tape in the player. Unfolding the poem, I peered down at the words. My knees buckled. The sheet of paper shook in my hands. This was tougher than I thought. In the movies, they made it look so easy.

The door opened, and in all her splendor, there stood Mary. A chill ran up my spine. In her left hand, she held a book. *She reads, she's perfect*, I thought. I took in a deep breath, reached down and pressed play. "Take My Breath Away" rang out; it was our song, our perfect song. I cleared my throat. At first I wanted to sing the poem, but Mary had a right to hear my voice, and a right to see my imperfections. My stuttering was interwoven into my being, and if she was going to love me, she had to love all of me. It's amazing how love—or in my case, infatuation—can become morphine to the soul, where fear and anxieties are numbed and one's vulnerability is exposed without any restraint. That was what happened to me when I decided to recite my poem accent-free, and with no safety net.

"Sh-Sh-e c-c-came f-f-f-from the c-c-c-clouds of h-h-heaven,
    Sh-Sh-She l-l-l-anded in my heart,
    I d-d-didn't know how b-b-b-beautiful she was
    Unt-t-t-til my heart sung l-l-like a harp."

Mary's hands covered her mouth. *Is she laughing? Is she in shock?* I reached into my backpack again, pulled out a bent rose and handed it to her.

"Thank you," she uttered. "I don't know what to say. I'm so flattered. No one has ever done this for me."

Grinning, I pressed the stop button. All was silent, nothing else had to be said. The moment would've been ruined by any more words that came out of my mouth. I grabbed my belongings, jumped on the bike and peddled off. I glanced behind me. Mary stood where I left her, watching me, waving at me, as her translucent smile brightened my way.

A week later, as the next CYO dance approached, my anticipation grew into fervor. Talking over my next bulletproof strategy with Pauley, it was clear that I was going to ask Mary to be my girlfriend at the dance. We would drift onto the dance floor as I sang a ballad in her ear. Our bodies would press together, and our hearts would beat to the same rhythm as she melted in my arms. She would love me forever. In the eyes of everyone—including the pair of eyes that looked back at me in the mirror every day—I would be a leading man.

Standing on the edge of the dance floor with Pauley, my eyes darted toward the double doors of the gymnasium as I caught site of her. Mary walked in with her rolled up jeans, flannel shirt, flowing hair, and her hand extended behind her.

I sprung into action, bounding my way toward her. The closer I got, the more I noticed whom she was holding onto. Her hand was interlaced with another guy's hand—a bigger guy with meat hook mitts and a sculpted physique. My heart sank as I took in the reality of it all. *This isn't how my movie ends.*

I heard Mary say something to me as I passed by them and out the door, but I ignored her; pride and shame muted any sound around me. Busting through the doors, I raced toward my house, leaving Pauley by himself. I didn't want him to know of my hurt. I already felt embarrassed.

Again, a woman had abandoned me and left me alone because I wasn't good enough, because I had this damn trembling voice that made me sound more like a head case than a passionate, perfect boy. Maybe if I recited the poem with fluency, or if my pudgy belly didn't flop over the sides of my pants, or if I was a little more dangerous, then maybe a beauty could love me.

The awkwardness and confusion gripped me, and I stopped in my tracks. The thought of going home ripped at my stomach. Facing Momma and Pop and having them ask me about my night at the dance would most assuredly send me into whirl of fury. Shame and isolation took the upper hand, and why should I break bad habits now?

Stopping at a set of iron gates that surrounded St. Benidle's playground, I wrenched on the metal barriers. I couldn't cry or lower myself into a comfortable sorrow. Rather, I chose a consolation prize, fortitude. This fortitude always derived from the same quandary: I just wanted to be heard. Why the hell couldn't I have that? Every human being deserved that right, the right to be understood and recognized. With each tug I gave on the gate, the harsh reality set in that I wasn't going to get everything I wanted. Many times I would stumble, fall, and break my neck for that small inch of victory, but was I willing to deal with the letdowns, pick myself up, and keep trying again?

20 The Theater Jargon

"I live halfway between reality and theater at all times."
—Lady Gaga

Disappointment became a normal facet to my life, and the more I perceived myself as the victim, the more I started to do the thing that would make any life coach cringe—I wallowed in self-pity. Without pushing forward and realizing that the reward lay in the effort instead of the end result, I remained at a standstill, scared to move and scared to take that next risk. Toward the beginning of my ninth grade at Rummel High, I lugged this complex around like a suitcase.

Distancing myself away from the CYO, the choir, and any other type of association with Mary gave me a sense of relief. Seeing Mary every Sunday would have been too uncomfortable—an unceasing reminder of my failure, and of the delusional certainty that a stuttering boy could attain love. Pauley understood why I had to quit singing at the Sunday services, and I was grateful for his support.

Outside of choir, Pauley and I continued our weekend excursions, but like most friendships entering their freshman year of high school, our relationship soon faded inconspicuously with no big hugs or tearful farewells. We just grew apart, never to pick up where we left off. To this day, I still cherish the times we spent together. Pauley helped me break free from some of my barriers and, like Sancho to my Quixote, encouraged me to battle the windmills beyond my reluctance.

Like most all-boy southern high schools, Rummel High's main interests were with football, baseball, swimming, and track and field. If you were a part of those four tiers, you were a demigod around campus. But I wasn't looking to be the next jock of the year. The arts called, and I had to take full advantage of whatever stutter-free and safe opportunities came my way, even if one of those opportunities included nine choirboys who were like me—the freaks and geeks of Rummel.

Through my freshman and sophomore year at Rummel, I dabbled in singing once again. The high I felt when crooning a song couldn't be ignored, and I had to reinstate singing back into my life. My asking to be in any choir was easier the second time around; and since most students weren't rushing in droves to Rummel's choir office begging and pleading to be a part of their unpopular club, the choir director—a portly priest who wore the pinkest skin I had ever seen—signed me up in an instant.

Activities with the choir involved being bused to retirement homes and singing for geriatrics, as well as rehearsing and performing for pep rallies and mass services. In time, my victimhood subsided, and I reveled in performing, which also came as a relief to my parents. This didn't mean I was ready to take on the role of Tom Cruise again or forget the discouragement from the Mary situation, but at least I was moving forward in my own secure—almost snail-like—pace.

In my nightly solitude as the bed sheets molded around my body, an entity continued to tug at me. It had no correlation with Momma Nettie or the guilt that still resided after her death. This internal entity was relentless, always reminding me that life had more to offer than better grades, choir practice, and other safe zones. Someone once told me when God provoked His children, He whispered. Well, if the Man upstairs was whispering to me all those nights—which I'm sure He was—one question lingered: Was I willing to abide to what He had to say?

Before long, a new opportunity seeped its way into my life when a wiry choir member named Jeff approached me with an unexpected prospect. Jeff had ushering duties for the upcoming play at Rummel, and because his grades were slipping, he couldn't partake in extra-curricular activities any longer, so it was his responsibility to find a replacement. Selling me on his offer, Jeff laid out the advantages of his ushering duties, which included free admission to the play, a foot in the door to the popular theater club at Rummel, and a chance to meet the director, Mr. Charles Guajardo—one of the most prominent high school theater directors in the city. My ushering chores involved cleaning the theater, handing out programs, and making sure people found their seats. With some hesitation, I agreed, thinking that if I involved myself in theater—which fascinated me to no end—then maybe I could satisfy the perpetual whisper in my head.

I had always possessed a yearning to be around the stage. Sure, I witnessed Sandy Duncan flying about, and I dabbled into the theatrics when I portrayed Herodias, or wore a Wiseman's gown, but to see my brother—someone from my world of suburbia—perform on a huge high school stage was something unprecedented. Between my fifth and eighth grade, I would faithfully attend my brother's theater performances at his high school—another influential all-boy high school that rivaled Rummel in every department, including theater. Attending plays ranging from *Arsenic & Old Lace*, to *Pippin*, I had my own theater appreciation class at my disposal as I sat in the front row, witnessing my brother do the very thing I could never accomplish. Studying each performance at least six or seven times with Momma, I would mouth the lines along with my brother as I lived vicariously through him. Though my brother would leave for college soon after, his performances stuck with me for years to come.

After his shows, my brother and his theater clique—which included young starry-eyed girls and boisterous over-the-top boys—gathered at our house, talking of the latest plays opening in New York, listening to musicals on vinyl, singing along with them, and doing impressions that left them howling in stitches. A bohemian group was thus conceived in our living room, and from an adjacent room, I would peek in and listen to their theater summits. Their critiques and banter about what constituted a good performance or a well-structured musical resonated with me. Soon a longing to be around the theater began to beat inside of my chest.

A couple of weeks after I agreed to take on Jeff's responsibilities, I found myself in the middle of what I had grown to adore. Ushering for Rummel's fall show—a heavy-duty courtroom drama called *Compulsions*—didn't feel like a chore at all; for me it was a privilege. After watching all twelve performances from the back of the sixty-seat house, I became an expert to Meyer Levin's play. For four weekends, I listened to the dialogue and how the actors changed their inflections from one night to the next. Like I did during my brother's performances, I quietly mouthed the words with the actors as I drank in the creative force radiating from the stage. My ears became attuned to a truthful moment when I heard one, and to a blasé delivery that sounded phony or canned.

Walking home after the performances, I would recite the lines, varying my tone and inflections. On those nightly walks where nothing else existed except the spoken words and the crisp air expanding my lungs, I promised myself that one day— one blessed day—I would step onto that stage. But for a stutterer, I envisioned myself as a torchbearer in *Man of La Mancha*, or an ensemble T-Bird in *Grease*. I could never be a lead. My impediment wouldn't allow such silly desires.

Asking for Saturdays off from Pop's auto shop was like asking him if I could drop out of school and join a cult. Ignoring Pop's indignation, Momma finally coerced my father into letting me spend my weekend mornings at Rummel's theater, where I helped tear down old sets, build new ones, position lights, and organize props. The grunt job—though not as glamorous as performing—gave me a deeper appreciation for theater. And no one in the theater group was impervious to getting his or her hands dirty. Even some of the leads from *Compulsions* were on their knees scraping off gum from under the house seats.

Over the hammering and the paint fumes in the air, I grew a fondness for the low-ceiling theater. Despite my eagerness to be around theater, I kept to myself, listening instead of talking, and studying others instead of engaging. The members who vigorously worked around me looked more like twenty-year olds than high school students, and I had never seen such a grand collection of pretty faces. I was somewhat intimidated by their appearances and the confidence they exuded, yet at the same time, I felt right at home. I was familiar with their airs of false security, their constant struggle for attention, and the theater jargon bouncing between them.

The Rummel Genesian Players—named after the patron saint of theater, St. Genesius—was formed in the late sixties by Charles Guajardo, infamously known as Mr. G. Short in height, but immense in personality, Mr. G. built Rummel's theater department from the ground up. As a child protégé who acted in a few Broadway plays, Mr. G. tried to sustain his youthful career in New York as he matured, but it seemed like the gods of theater wanted him remembered as a kid actor instead of an adult actor. With his chances limited in having a flourishing career, Mr. G. moved to New Orleans, where he found a more prosperous career in teaching. He landed a job at Rummel, married, had two daughters, created The Genesian Players, built a playhouse on campus, and touched hundreds of lives through the everlasting language of theater.

The first words Mr. G. ever imparted to me happened on a random Saturday morning. With a coffee in his left hand, he approached me, "I've been seeing you around here, but we never had the pleasure."

Extending his wide hand toward me, he introduced himself, "I'm Mr. G., and you are...?"

"Scott," I replied. No stutter occurred, for I had rehearsed that response many times before.

"Well, welcome." And with that simple introduction, Mr. G. left me to my hammering and sweating. Studying his walk as he crossed the stage, I noticed his stubby legs and his long arms dramatically waving back and forth. He had poise and style about his demeanor, mirroring a dancer's physique as he swaggered with grace. His tawny skin glowed like he just walked off a tropical island. He had an air of confidence that could not be ignored. Intimidating, yet accessible at the same time, Mr. G. seemed as if he always carried valuable information locked away under his salt and pepper hair. For some ungodly reason, my life seemed a little more enriched after I met my future high school mentor, even though I didn't know why at the time. I'd find out soon enough.

21 Ensemble No More

"If you go in and audition for roles rather than just be offered them, then you kind of get a chance to kind of discover that you can do something that you didn't think you could do."
—Peter Sarsgaard

In the spring of my sophomore year, as I scurried down the hall to make it to my Monday morning class, a pink flyer grabbed my attention. I ignored it, but like cologne, it followed me around all day. Every corner I turned, similar flyers dangled from the various bulletin boards around campus, taunting and begging me to read its bold fonts. Giving in, I pulled one off its tack.

"The Genesian Players proudly announces upcoming auditions for their production of *Little Shop of Horrors*. Saturday afternoon at 1 P.M."

Reading it twice over, I couldn't believe my eyes. An optimistic pulsation rang through me. For months, I had waited patiently for the right show and the right moment to audition for The Genesian Players. According to the pink flyer in my hand, the moment had finally arrived.

Among the many musicals my brother blasted throughout the house, *Little Shop of Horrors* was one of those recurring recordings that landed on my ears. In due time, I sang along with the catchy tunes from the popular Ashman and Menken musical, as my involuntary attention to the soundtrack turned into my greatest pleasure. After a while, I could sing any *Little Shop* song from memory. But five years later, in February 1989, the stakes were higher, and I wondered if I still knew the musical by heart.

With the flyer in hand, I rushed home and snuck into my brother's room. Everything stayed the way he had left it since he returned to NYU for his second year of college. Flipping through his record collection, I came upon it—a green record jacket with the illustration of a horrific plant devouring a blonde damsel. Slipping the vinyl from its sleeve, I placed the record on my brother's player, pressed the needle down, and sang with the recording as if a day hadn't passed. An air of relief filled the room when I realized I could still sing the musical backwards and forwards as Ellen Green and I harmonized "Suddenly Seymour."

When I decided I wanted to audition for Rummel's production of *Little Shop*, my sights were set on a chorus role. I had grown accustomed to being in the background because my stuttering unfailingly cast me in that role. As the audition approached, I planned the whole scenario in my head; I was going to articulate my ensemble interest to Mr. G., sing my heart out, and then leave as quickly as coming in, nothing else to prove or gamble. Knowing that singing was my strong suit, I had every intention of blowing the director away with my prepared ballad.

With certainty at my heels, I walked onto the stage that Saturday afternoon and looked out, somewhat blinded by the stage lights pointing down at me.

"And what are you singing for us today, Scott?" asked Mr. G. as his silhouette leaned forward in the back row.

" 'Sudd-d-denly Seymour,' " I answered.

"Good!" barked Mr. G. "Carry on, then."

Being on the Genesian stage for the first time, I felt a sudden chill run up my spin, but this sensation didn't derive from a place of fear or apprehension. On the contrary, I felt right at home, and I think that's what jarred me the most.

Clearing my throat, I sang the song a cappella. I didn't need an accompanist; I knew every inflection, and every riff by heart as my gestures waved and flapped with reason. In my mind, I pictured Momma Nettie in that last row, looking on and smiling as I sang for her. I let her memory drive me through the song. If this was my first introduction to method acting, I wasn't privy to it at the time.

With cordial decorum to his voice, the silhouetted Mr. G. raised his hand and graciously stopped me midway. Fidgeting, I waited impatiently for Mr. G.'s verdict. It seemed like an hour, yet only thirty seconds had passed when I heard him say, "I'd like to hear you read for Seymour. Could you grab sides outside and come back in an hour?"

He said that unforgiving word...sides!

In the "biz," sides refer to pages of dialogue that are used during auditions. They can either include pages of various scenes or just four or five lines on one page. Sides are utilized so the director — and whoever else is in the room — can hear the actor in a particular role. Usually, there are two characters interacting within the sides, sometimes three. It is customary for actors to receive sides well in advance so that they can properly prepare. These sides can be an actor's greatest tool or worst nightmare when auditioning. In that tiny theater, I felt the latter, especially when Mr. G's impromptu request was thrust upon me.

My knees buckled while my mouth wanted to yell in protest, "No, please, I just want to be a chorus boy!" But I censored myself. I didn't want disappoint the unwavering Mr. G. or show any signs of weakness. If he asked me to read sides, I'd oblige, even if it meant humiliation.

For half an hour and with no one around, I read the lines over and over again out loud to the point of memorization. In my isolated spot — which happened to be an adjacent hall — the lines gushed out of my mouth without a stutter. Elocution came when I read by myself, but what I expected to unfold in front of Mr. G., his assistant, and his reader would probably be a contrasting scenario. I'd have listening ears and deciding eyes scrutinizing my delivery, as the bad no-no's would most certainly paralyze my tongue. For sure I was going to stammer like an idiot in front of strangers; and I already accepted the lie that I had told myself many times before.

Once they called out my name, I shuffled slowly to the theater. Anxiety-ridden thoughts galloped through my mind. Maybe if I just explained to Mr. G. that I didn't want the role, then he would excuse me. Yes, that would be the easiest way out, but was I being honest with myself and to the Godly voice that still crept into my bedroom? How badly did I want this? Without invitation, Ross swung his way to the forefront of my mind—the baker who had no regrets, no excuses, and no intentions to live in the shadow of his dysfunction. If I wanted to play with the big boys, I had to live the life that Ross represented. If I hungered to make an appearance on stage, I had to hurl myself into the fear, and let the victimhood take a vacation, even for a little while. I owed that much to myself.

As Mr. G. led me into the theater and asked if I had any questions about the material, a tactic came to mind. I decided to summon a dialect that paralleled the actor from the original recording—who sounded more like Woody Allen than anything else. With the limited time I had between walking into the theater and taking the stage, I preoccupied myself more with creating a character than letting my stuttering dictate a dismal fate. As always, my imagination swooped in and saved me. Determined to do the unthinkable, I was going to give the sides a whirl.

Mr. G. took his place at the back of the house. On stage, the female reader smiled and nodded at me.

"Whenever you're ready," she said in a hush.

She was a striking blonde, with glowing blue eyes. Her beauty was distracting, and I couldn't look at her for too long. Glaring at the pages, I took in a deep breath. I felt my diaphragm tighten as I muttered my first line toward the female reader. The Yiddish-Brooklyn accent was placed perfectly in my mouth:

Seymour: "Oh A-Audrey, you're the most wonderful p-person that ever lived. We're gonna get that l-little house and everything's gonna be alright, you'll see."

I got the first line out of the gate, and with that, I succumbed to an unmatched serenity. The accent and the character recall propelled me forward, and both armed me with certitude as I threw the sides to the ground. I knew the material, and it was mine to be had. Continuing on, I pieced the words, phrases, and heightened emotions together. To my delight, my slight stammers lent to Seymour Krelborn's nervousness and high-tension. All those times of constant imitations, mimicking, and impersonations were finally paying off. *Christ, wouldn't Raphael be so proud!*

"Very good, very, very good," Mr. G. whispered as we ended the scene. He walked down the five steps and onto the stage. I looked to my co-star who gave me an encouraging wink, a similar wink I had received two years prior from a brunette in a church.

"Can you come back tomorrow?" Mr. G. asked. "I want to hear you sing with our musical director."

The following day, in the petite theater, I belted out two songs from the show I already knew from memory. The musical director asked me if I needed any sheet music, to which I politely responded with a no thank you. This may have seemed cocky on my end, but I knew performing without sheet music or pages of dialogue freed me up, alleviated the tension from stuttering, and gave me more room to play...and play I did. As the musical director pounded away at the keyboards, I slid and glided on each note like a surfer on a perfect wave. I crooned "Grow For Me" with zeal.

Later that week, Mr. G. called to inform me that I would be double cast as Seymour Krelborn, which meant I would share the role with another actor. Lighting had struck twice, once at Christian Brothers, and now with Mr. G.'s offer. Hanging up the phone after profusely thanking Mr. G., I darted to the kitchen. I couldn't wait to tell Momma and Pop they had another actor in their house.

But before I reached the kitchen, I slowed my pace. The party in my head ceased as an uncertainty took over my revelry: What if I couldn't pull off this charade during rehearsals and my violent stuttering made a cameo appearance? Like a newly designed car, I had yet to prove the successful longevity of my accent usage. Was I doomed for disaster? Only time would tell...and a whole lotta prayer.

22 A Kiss That Sailed a Thousand Performances

"The truth needs so little rehearsal."
—Barbara Kingsolver

"You're gonna make a fool of yourself, and I can't watch you do that."

Momma didn't say these exact words to me, yet I heard her reservations every time I caught her staring at me while I rehearsed my lines, or during dinner when I recounted what happened that day at play practice. Momma's worrisome eyes, furrowed brow, and the downward arch to her mouth said it all. Aware of her telltale responses, she would quickly force an affable smile, holding back any remarks that could quite possibly cut me to the core. As the mother of a stutterer, how could she not have some semblance of doubt?

In his usual style, Pop wasn't as subtle with his lack of encouragement. His practical, old-fashioned mindset got in the way of supporting my stage debut. "Great, another goddamn actor in the house," and "He should be at the shop and not flittin' around some stage," were the usual grumbles I'd overhear rolling out of Pop's mouth. But I paid no heed to his comments. In fact, their pessimism propelled me forward during those first weeks of rehearsals. The more they heaped their misgivings upon me, the more Pop's words ricocheted in my head—"Life ain't cheap. A man has to pay a price to get what he wants"— the more I was determined to use Pop's own advice to prove him wrong.

To my surprise, the first week of rehearsals—which included learning music with the musical director, rehearsing the dance numbers that Mr. G. choreographed, and blocking out the scenes on stage—were absent of any hitches. During those initial weeks, I didn't have to concern myself with lines. So far, everything was going swimmingly, and the cast couldn't have been more supportive of one another.

Every principal role was double cast, and Mr. G.'s reason for doing so was to help the actors rest their voices, as well as give ample opportunities for more students to appear in meatier roles. Because I shared the role with another actor—a young, ambitious actor who was a year older than I—a mild calmness set in when I realized the responsibility to carry the show didn't just lay on my shoulders. Brick had been in a couple of the Genesian plays, and *Little Shop* marked his third lead role at Rummel. Well aware of his résumé and his thunderous voice onstage, Brick carried himself with confidence, but he never threw any reproachful remarks my way. We would exchange hellos, acknowledge each other's presence with a few pleasantries, and observe one another's performances. Perhaps I had an acquired taste for his alpha personality, which had a striking resemblance to my brother's temperament. Nevertheless, a healthy competitiveness grew between Brick and I, and the grand prize—ultimately decided by the great arbitrator, Mr. G.—would be who performed on opening night.

The more I watched Brick's rehearsals from the back of the theater, the more I felt inferior to his onstage charisma. Eventually, this insecurity pushed me harder to be the best Seymour Krelborn the school had ever seen, and to not succumb to the stuttering, which usually ran alongside my timidities. In doing so, I rigorously studied my lines and crafted my accent. Like my audition, I discovered the stammering was kept at a minimum when off book.

Attempting to keep my impediment a secret offstage, I made sure I didn't converse as much with fellow cast members. I had developed a knack for asking simple questions and letting others rant about themselves. With theater folk, this strategy was

an easy task to accomplish, which lent to my reputation as the
new kid who sported a smile, listened attentively, came to
rehearsals off book, and was fully vested in his role. But little did
the cast know that every time I entered the theater, hesitation
trailed right behind me. According to my warped sense of
reality, if I exposed any remnants of my dysfunction, Mr. G.
would let Brick take over the role solely, and thus ending my
short-lived acting career. To say a self-inflicted pressure was
percolating inside of me would've been an understatement.

Within that month and a half of rehearsals, I had a crash
course in theater etiquette. From how to come fully prepared to
rehearsals, how to take direction, and the meaning of crossing
downstage, upstage, stage left, and stage right, Mr. G. shared his
years of knowledge with us. With his wealth of experience came
an unrelenting discipline from him.

"Is that the best choice you can come up with?" was a usual
rhetorical question he asked when the line didn't come from an
honest place. Another common phrase Mr. G. bellowed out was,
"Do you know how many people wanted this role? You better
bring your A game if you want to be in here!"

His imperious manner unnerved me quite a bit. I would
sweat like a pig every time I fouled up or when I heard a
grumble come from his silhouetted figure in the last row. But I
sucked in deep breaths, calmed my nerves and stuck to the
words and accent. To my surprise, being onstage was easier than
being off; at least onstage I could manipulate my voice and hide
behind a well-rehearsed character.

Sooner than I thought, one of my worst fears came into
fruition as Mr. G. caught on to my stuttering. It happened a
couple of weeks before opening. During that time, I felt the
fatigue creeping in, and the charade to be the perfect boy was
growing tiresome. Added to the mix was Momma and Pop's
unrelenting doubt in my outcome. I tried to push these
unproductive factors to the back of my head, but like an
avalanche, they all came tumbling down once I started stuttering

on stage. Bad severe, clicking sounds arose on stage as well as the paraphrasing of lines, the sprinkling of buffers into the dialogue, and the replacing of written words with my own safe words.

After his patience had hit an end, Mr. G. yelled out, "That's not what's on the page, Scott! If you're going to learn your lines, learn them correctly!"

Perhaps Mr. G. sensed something in my sullen look and how I was on the brink of tears. But after I excused myself for a moment, Mr. G. followed me into the hall and asked if I was having trouble with the material.

I lied, "N-No, sir."

"Then why are you paraphrasing? Don't you know we have to respect the author's words?"

I nodded, and realized the jig was up. I had no other alternative but to tell Mr. G. that I was a stutterer. After I laid it out for him, a long pause followed; like in the plays he directed, Mr. G. had a knack for creating long dramatic pauses.

I broke the silence, "P-Please, d-don't' t-take me out of the p-play."

He patted me on the shoulder, gave the warmest smile I had ever seen from him, and walked away. As he stepped out of the hallway, I heard him say, "I'll see you back on stage in ten. We have work to do." He didn't give me time to feel sorry for myself.

After my chat with Mr. G., my acting became sharper. I didn't have to keep my dark secret hidden from him any longer. He knew, I knew, and now we could forge ahead. As a result, I found my onstage instincts more organic and more truthful. I had a freer reign to my movements and to my character, all because I told Mr. G. I wasn't perfect. In time, an astonishing revelation came to me as I was forced to look at my dysfunction from a different perspective. Because I exhaustingly tried to impress others and strived to be the best son, actor, student, and boy for everyone, my body reacted by creating a tension in how I spoke. Giving others power as well as giving into the farcical quest for perfection came at a hefty cost. Yet when I did things for me, to just enjoy them, and when I had a comfortable, calm, and confident demeanor on stage—some would call it "being in the zone"—where I forgot about Scott and became a living, breathing character, that was when I would hammer away at words with elocution.

My attraction to theater wasn't just because I envisioned myself as being adored and accepted by everyone; theater was a gateway to leave my inhibitions far behind me. In turn, I morphed into a beloved character, and found a sacred part of me—a better, perfect side of me that the playwright allowed me to express. Within that realm between reality and fantasy, I could forgo all of my worries and allow myself to speak like a normal person.

A week before our premiere, the opening night cast was announced. To my elation, and to Brick's disappointment, I would be performing in the opening cast. After his announcement, Mr. G. gave me the reason behind his choice, "It wasn't out of pity I chose you, Scott. You earned it."

On opening night, the jitters yanked my insides. I paced around like a chicken with his head cut off, reviewing my lines out loud in the solitude of the hallway. I could hear the audience's mutters coming from the theater. Any minute I would step onto the Genesian stage in front of an eager crowd, which also included my parents.

That was when she approached me, the dance captain named Karen who was almost two years my senior, who was more developed than any seventeen year-old-girl I had ever met and who, like a sonnet, moved and glided gracefully on and offstage. While I mostly listened, Karen and I shared many conversations about her family, their strict discipline, and how dance consumed her life. But our conversations weren't too deep or earth shattering. Knowing that Karen was way out of my league, I never thought she could have any interest in a stutterer.

At fifteen, I didn't pick up on her subtle hints like my name scribbled in her notebook with a heart behind it, or her incessantly asking me if I needed a ride home. The lack of security that came with my stuttering blinded me from the obvious.

"You're going to be great," Karen said in a hesitant tone. Her eyes shifted, and she fidgeted with her costume dress, compulsively stringing her fingers along the hem. Before I had the chance to deduce why the hell she was so nervous, she planted a kiss on me; a full body kiss that released any type of tension I had in my mouth and throat. After gently pulling away, she whispered, "I'm so proud of you."

She then passed by me like a peaceful breeze and was gone. Not wanting to forget the poignant moment that had just transpired, I froze, unable to move. I had never felt such exaltation in my body. Suddenly, courage started to build inside of me. Steadfast and undaunted, I was ready to make my debut on stage. I was going to knock them dead, because a beauty told me so.

Making my way to the backstage, I reflected on Karen's words. There was something in her cadence that felt like home. I could've sworn I heard remnants of Momma Nettie in Karen's uplifting words. As I walked to my place in the wings, I felt my great-grandmother in me and all around me. Taking in deep soothing breaths, I could've sworn I smelled the scent of Salem's and Scotch tickling my nose.

23 The Leading Man

There's something about the thunder bursting from applauding hands that gives a performer a taste of eternity. When you take that final bow, the cheers pulsating through your soul make you feel like Poseidon ruling over the great seas. But when a stutterer hears the applause, it is more than just a rapturous sensation. It is like dying and entering Elysian Fields.

As the drenched costume clung to me, and the overuse of my voice tingled in the back of my throat, I took my first bow before a standing ovation. I was fatigued from the two and a half hour show, but the exhaustion didn't matter once I heard the resounding applause. Whooping and hollering, the audience represented the epitome of graciousness. Accepting the accolades with the cast as we bowed a third time, I finally had a chance to reflect on my performance.

During the performance, I didn't stumble once. Forgoing any hesitation, I blocked out the stuttering and was in the zone for what seemed like a marathon. My voice was in tack, and nothing distracted me from the job at hand. I felt Seymour in me—his accent, his walk, and his objective firmly driving me to my goal. The audience's attentiveness fueled me further as I delivered an almost flawless performance.

After the curtain call, the cast and audience convened at the opening night gala, which reflected a festive mood—hugs, warm accolades, and fellow cast members exclaiming, "We did it!" over and over again like manic patients. Even though I appreciated the celebratory energy of the party and the irresistible attention I was getting from Karen, all I wanted to do was find my parents and see the pride exuding from their faces. Ducking and weaving my way through the packed party, I finally caught up with them. Momma was the first to embrace me. "My God, how'd you learn all those lines?" she asked.

I noticed a certain spark radiating from her green eyes—a tranquil and positive expression I had been waiting months to witness. Years later, Momma would confess just how relieved she had been to see her boy perform successfully in front of a live audience. Numerous times leading up to opening night, she had picked up the phone, ready to call Mr. G. and discuss my stuttering, and the disaster that would ensue if I appeared on stage. She wanted to talk him out of his casting choice, and maybe coerce him into putting me in a minor role. Like any concerned mother, Momma didn't want to witness her son collapsing from the pressure and the laughs that came with the stammering. Once again, she would have to pick up the pieces, and I guess Momma's heart had no more to give in that arena. Call it God's unseen hand holding her finger back, or Momma's faith in me superseding her overprotective nature, but something stopped her from dialing that last digit. To this day, I am eternally grateful she never dialed Mr. G.'s number. At least her coddling knew some boundaries.

Embracing Pop in the middle of the reception, I felt my father pat my shoulders as he said, "That was good acting there. You got good stuff." He diverted his eyes, and his lips morphed into a tight smile. I could tell Pop wanted to tell me something more, but he held back.

The play ran for four weekends, and I performed Seymour every other night, even though the exhilaration I experienced on opening night couldn't be topped. Thereafter, every time I said a word or phrase on stage without stumping, stammering, or replacing words, a silent celebration ignited within me. Never again would I take such simple undertakings lightly.

Repetition with the material had become a valuable asset. It helped me solidify my intentions on stage and build a confidence in my voice. The more I performed, the more I discovered nuances and deliveries that derived from a deeper part of me. Not one performance was ever the same as the next. Never phoning it in, I felt myself connected with Seymour, and soon we were viscerally synonymous. I yearned to hit the pause button and have my life stay at a standstill, forever feeling the rapture that stage acting brought to my life. But as they say in show business, two things are always certain: Shows open and shows close.

On closing night, as I packed up my belongings and made my way out of the dressing room, Mr. G. stopped me in my tracks, shook my hand firmly, pointed toward the theater, and said, "Don't forget this. Ever."

And I wouldn't.

How could I forget the feeling of invincibility and triumph that unrivaled anything I had ever accomplished? But before long, I had to relinquish the world of Seymour Krelborn and return to the realm I detested the most—Scott's world.

Days following closing night, Karen distracted me from my post-show blues by delving into a committed relationship with me. But our young inexperienced affair wasn't mature enough to fill an uncertain void that germinated within me. Affiliated with this void was a reminder that maybe my life in theater was a one-time deal. Every fiber of my being wanted to get back onto the stage and prove to no one else but myself that *Little Shop* wasn't a fluke. But Genesian's next season didn't start till September, and we were entering the first weeks of summer. Three months separated me and my next opportunity to feel like a normal stutter-free boy, and even then, I wasn't promised a role. Instead of days spent living in the skin of a character and in a story that was bigger than me, I found myself floundering and sweating six days a week at Pop's shop.

My restlessness and skepticism about my future filtered into my work at the shop. Instead of answering the phone with,

"Hello, auto service. How may I help you?" — a professional greeting Pop demanded of everyone — I'd replace my greeting with, "Y-Y-Yes?" When my days were filled with rehearsing and performing, I could execute such undertakings like answering a phone or ordering take-out with minor stammers. But now I had given up, never striving for elocution in my real life. If I didn't have the stage, what was the point in trying? Soon Pop caught on to my replacement greeting, and banned me from answering the phone altogether. Once again, I felt like a failure.

Everything in me felt uneasy and monotonous, and as the erosion of my confidence hit a tipping point, I tried to immerse myself in other artistic endeavors — reading more, sketching more, going to the movies with Karen and talking about the film's message. But like an uninvited drunk uncle coming to Christmas dinner, the victimhood crept back into my psyche and resided there for a while, never allowing me to enjoy life with my new girlfriend.

Tattooing an artificial grin on my face, I never shared my ever-increasing tension and doubt with anyone, especially with Karen. I didn't want her to think I was broken or imperfect. To hide my disappointments, I fixated on another manufactured role, a self-manifested charade I would later call "The Leading Man Syndrome."

Besides earning a vocal confidence during *Little Shop* performances, I developed a more grievous identity complex when performing onstage. Related to co-dependency, this syndrome entailed a delusion of grandeur that said if I could display my perfections onstage in lead roles, then — like a packaged toy — I would become a wanted commodity offstage without anyone noticing my inadequacies. And who could walk away from me then? Instead of others concentrating on my damaged voice in the real world, they would accept me for the person they perceived on stage — I could be their Ralph Macchio or Tom Cruise. In turn, I would be the perfect specimen, saving anyone from their problems, as I concealed my own flaws.

With Karen came an intimidating factor and, according to my distorted perspective, she could never love a stutterer. So I pressed this leading man syndrome into fourth gear by creating a visceral production where I would be the center of attention in Karen's world. On my subconscious stage, I would save her from the pressures that came with her family life, or any type of insecurities that were synonymous with her being a performer. If I had to relinquish my leading man role in *Little Shop,* I sure as hell wasn't going to let go of my leading man persona in my personal life.

As the summer days rolled along in 1989, my neediness turned to obsession when it came to Karen. I'd relentlessly call her, asking when I could see her, or when she could drive me to the movie theater so we could forget ourselves for a little while. Putting such a burden on someone's shoulders was too much to ask from anyone and ultimately, Karen became irritated when I pointed out her flaws instead of my own, and the desperate pleas that came out of me, "W-Where are you?" "I n-n-need you so much," and "W-We'll be t-together forever." Little did I know, I was slowly sabotaging our relationship and writing the ending that was most comfortable for me — the leading woman exiting stage left.

Towards the end of the summer, Karen performed at the prestigious Tulane Summer Lyrics Festival — a musical theater festival featuring popular musicals with out-of-town guest artists in the lead. Karen was cast as a featured dancer in the festival's season closer, *Evita.* For a high school student going into her senior year, Karen was given a unique opportunity to work alongside some of the most talented professionals in the city.

Her involvement in the Summer Lyrics meant less time with her "Scotty," and as a result, a little resentment built up inside of me. I felt like a supporting role in the production called *Karen & Scott,* and my pride and insecurities couldn't allow such a casting choice. Stubbornly, I was going to fight for her attention. She needed me, or so my fears dictated.

On opening night of *Evita*, I made sure Momma dropped me off an hour earlier so I could grab a perfect seat in the theater. I sat in the middle second row as I tightly held a bouquet of flowers. That night she performed exquisitely, every straight line and every breathless move executed. She was a sight to behold.

In the crowded backstage hallway, which led to the dressing rooms, I darted toward Karen. Nearing, I noticed a tall older gentleman leaning in and whispering into Karen's ear. He sported a soul patch like a beatnik poet. Showing off his perfect physique, this Kerouac-wannabe had his jacket unbuttoned, exposing his hairy chest. Instantly I recognized him as the actor who played the lead. Karen giggled at his whispered comment as she slapped his chest in a flirtatious way, like they were old chums.

"Hey, b-babe," I said, interrupting their interlude.

She bolted upright from her comfortable state as if she was caught doing something wrong. Thinking nothing of it, I congratulated her and handed her the flowers. I tried to make eye contact with the older gentleman, but somehow he couldn't look me directly in the eyes. An uncomfortable feeling swirled between the three of us. I broke the awkwardness by extending my hand out to the stranger, "H-Hi, I'm Scott."

He met me with a limp wrist handshake. Karen introduced us. "This is Darin. He's an actor from Los Angeles. He's here as a guest artist."

He managed a pretentious "Ciao," and then he was off, probably bee-lining his way to some other impressionable girl. Clearing her throat, Karen gave me an unhappy look, as if I was intruding or cramping her style. "Look, we're going to a bar to celebrate our opening. I mean, I'd ask you to come, but you don't have an ID, and well...I didn't want to miss hanging out with the cast..." Karen had a fake ID. I didn't. She was always ahead of the game.

Playing the understanding boyfriend, I told Karen to go, have fun, and that I would call Momma to come pick me up.

Waiting outside of the theater, I reflected on my absurd predicament. Like she had so many times before, my mother was about to pick me up in the Malibu Classic, while my girlfriend was driving herself to some undisclosed bar with the big boys, with a real leading man, with Darin. My life was on pause. Karen's life was on fast forward.

The shocking, yet inevitable letter soon followed — the usual, "I'm sorry, I hope we can be friends" letter that accompanies any type of break-up. In the two-page note, Karen talked about how she needed to lead the life she wanted, not one where she had to constantly please everyone around her. Then she dropped a huge bomb that imploded in my heart. "I am moving with Darin to Los Angeles. I want to be a dancer out there and even though you and my parents may not support me in this decision, I must take it."

Crumpling the letter, I threw it to the side. I didn't want to hold it anymore. Reading it reminded me of who I really was — a chorus boy, a minor role, an ensemble. No one could love a buffoon like me, a stammering idiot who could never be a leading man for any girl, not for Mary, not for Karen, not for any type of fantasy girl. It was easier to stick solo and to commit myself to the only lady who made me feel whole.

24 The Notebooks

My breakup with Karen propelled me into another romantic interlude, but this relationship was with a female who had no gender, no physical attributes, and no mortality. I began my junior year committing every waking moment to this ethereal being. She gave back more than anyone in my life, and calmed the inner turmoil this stutterer hauled around day in and day out. She built me up, but she knew how to tear me down just the same. Hook, line and sinker, I was hers for the taking. Theater was her name.

For the next two years, I plunged into the world of drama—stage construction, rehearsals, learning lines and beats, and authenticating dialects that hid my impaired voice. With my involvement in the theater club, Karen turned into a distant memory, yet the pang from the breakup still remained. Silencing the abandonment, I distracted myself by plunging into any role Mr. G. deemed fit for me to portray. If I continued my appearances onstage and had an outlet to express myself, I was less inclined to share my grievances with Momma and Pop about not fitting in as a stutterer, about the uncertainty of what I wanted to do once I graduated, and the concern about whether a girl would ever date me again. The less secure I felt, the more I dedicated every minute to theater. Eventually, I found myself pretending more in my real life than onstage.

The Genesian Theater soon became my home away from home. From my small role as the diner owner in the dark drama *When Ya Comin' Back, Red Rider*, to the slick-back, smart ass Kenickie in *Grease*, various parts came my way, mostly minor or supporting roles, but hardly the lead. According to my ego, it didn't matter whether I had a few lines or a two-page monologue, I wanted to be near that tangible vapor called The Arts, which reminded me that I still had something to say and a way to say it.

Besides my complicated emotions, some areas in my life did seem less challenging, especially when auditioning for Mr. G. Always off book and always performing with a dialect, I knew the space and what to expect when I entered the Genesian Theater. Familiarizing myself with the material and masking behind a character were my greatest allies in the war against stuttering, and this preparation seemed to please Mr. G. to no end. It was a win-win situation for both of us.

As my obsession for escapism developed, I became more involved with other theater clubs in the area, especially all-girl schools where male actors were in high demand. Sometimes I'd juggle two plays at one time. When one play opened, I'd jump right into rehearsals for the other. From a hillbilly to an English professor, I evolved into the ultimate chameleon. Because of my look and the plays that I selected to be a part of, I was cast in roles that required an accent. Call it luck, a sub-conscience manifestation, or maybe the Big Casting Director in the sky was looking out for me. Whatever the reason, I had become a character actor as I neared the end of my high school career.

When I walked into an audition for the other schools, I never introduced myself with my real voice. Relying on my tricks of the trade, I was certain the stuttering would come out since they didn't know my potential on stage. Believing that no one like Mr. G. would ever take a chance with a stutterer, I remained in character throughout the whole audition. Like David Copperfield, I gave them the grand illusion.

Compared to dating or interacting with girls, I found performing in roles easier feats. I had more confidence onstage with females than I did offstage with them. When I had to tell a girl, "I love you" under the beams of a spotlight, it was less messy, and less challenging. But the thought of dating in real life, or telling a girl how

I felt about her rattled me with fear. Sure, I had pretty, attractive, and talented girls around me, and I harbored unsaid crushes, but I never pursued them, and never ventured forth to ask if she wanted to go to the movies, or go to a late-night grub fest at the local Friday's. Sooner or later, girls ran away from me, cheated on me, or died on me. Stutterers always lost on that playing field, but not in theater, not in the art of make-believe. I knew the ending when I just stuck to the script.

It wasn't long before my brother heard about my ventures in theatre. Returning home in January of 1990, my brother found me in the living room pouring over my lines for one of my upcoming shows. "Mom tells me you're doing plays."

I nodded, feeling his judgmental stare pressing down on me.

He raised an arched smile as I looked up. "But you know you have to have proper training to make it a career," he said firmly, effecting a Standard English accent he'd developed during his studies abroad. "You can't just look at it as a hobby. But for you it'll always be a hobby, right?"

I didn't answer. I'd lose the argument if I even attempted to stand up for myself. My brother's quick tongue always beat me to the punch. Rather, I returned to my lines, quietly seething.

I didn't want to admit it at the time, but my brother had a valid point, and why wouldn't I heed his words of caution? He had almost four years under his belt in New York, and in that time, he'd studied under some of the best instructors in theater, directed a play for Tish School of the Arts, studied a semester in England, and had set his sights on staying in New York to pursue an acting career. As the days followed, his imparting words lay heavily on my heart. If I wanted to make a career out of acting and not as a coping hobby or a means to forget myself, then I'd have to look at it more as a vocation than anything else.

Usually when my brother visited home, most of his time involved catching up with old friends from his former bohemian group. Since I hadn't seen much of him during that particular winter break, I thought it would be a safe bet to enter my brother's room, rummage through his notes from class, and do a little thespian research without his knowledge. To pursue a career in theater, I'd have to find out what the hell I was getting into. Keeping most of his life a secret by hiding behind an astute exterior, my brother hardly shared his knowledge about his craft, or any deep insight regarding his emotions. He always held the advantage that way.

Taking the initiative by entering his closed off lair, I entered his room and opened his closet. In the corner, below some old sweaters and jackets, I found a taped up brown box. On the side, it said, "Notes."

With a delicate touch, I peeled back the thick layer of tape and opened the box. What I found inside were a treasure of stacked notebooks; all labeled "class notes." They were my brother's notes from the past four years. My hand shook in excitement as I reached down, grabbed the first notebook from the top and flipped it open. On top of the first scribbled page was an archaic letterhead that had inked stars and five lines drawn underneath its lettering, "Stella Adler's Class. Fall '88."

My eyes felt as if they were about to pop out of their sockets. In my hands were the detailed notes from one of the most acclaimed drama teachers in the history of theater. Stella Adler — a known tyrant and an avid follower of the Stanislavsky technique — was a preeminent acting teacher whose apprentices included Robert DeNiro and Marlon Brando. I had heard of her from the countless books I'd read on the history of acting as well as the biographies of celebrities. Now at my disposal were Adler's dictated words, which were written down in my brother's chicken scratch penmanship.

Time whisked by as I carefully read from the notebook, delving deeper into my true passion. To my astonishment, most of what Adler preached paralleled Mr. G. teachings — embodying the truth onstage and having every word come from an organic source based on the character, as well as the author's intentions.

Nearing the end of the third or fourth notebook, I suddenly felt a pinch of guilt. My intentions on stage were real, but not my voice.

Was I going against the greats? Were my accents limiting my full potential for truth on stage? What would happen if I used my real voice?

The hours passed as I finished one notebook and grabbed another. All that mattered were the notes, the lessons I wanted to put into action, and the gentle whisper in my ear telling me that this profession of words, emotions, and heightened awareness might encompass my future.

Suddenly, the tugging of the closet door made me jump out of my skin. There above me—with a petulant look to his face—was my brother. Resembling Pop's pursed lips every time he was angry, my brother's lips tightened as he stared down at me. But unlike Pop, my brother said what he thought without a filter, "You barbaric ass! What are you doing to my belongings?" Since studying in England, my brother frequently injected Shakespearean euphemisms whenever he was volatile. This annoyed my family and I to no end.

Unaware of my present surroundings, I realized most of his notebooks were strewn all about me. My hand was in the cookie jar. I had been caught red-handed. There was no hiding it. "I-I-I'm sorry. I-I-I..."

My brother cut me off. "I don't care! You're not supposed to touch these! These are irreplaceable! I will not have them marred!"

Like an archaeologist picking up rare artifacts, my brother gently grabbed his notebook and placed them in the box. Once he got closer to me, he shouted, "Get out! Just don't step on the pearls!" "Pearls" were in reference to his notebooks.

I followed most of his commands, but instead of leaving the room, I sat on the edge of his bed until he finished organizing his belongings. I wanted to explain myself further, "I-I-I was just r-reading them. I-I was going to p-put them b-back." I was certain he would tattle, and my parents would reprimand me, prohibiting me from ever entering his room.

My brother swiveled around and faced me. "You don't know anything about acting. And even if you wanted to, you couldn't with your..." He pointed to his mouth, rudely referring to the unsaid.

My hands clenched the bedspread. I felt the heat sinking from my shoulders to my arms. My instincts screamed at me to leap up and pound the crap out of him. Instead, I remained on the bed, listening to the abuse unfolding in front of me.

"Stick with your drawings. You're good at that, but not this. You can't be an actor." And with that last stinging comment, my brother pressed his hand on my back and led me to his door. Shrugging his hand from off of me, I walked out of the room, trying to shut out my brother's piercing condemnations.

25 The Last Hurrah-Rah

"No man was ever great by imitation."
—Samuel Johnson

My brother's repressive comments stayed with me for quite some time, escalating the self-doubt that resided in my relationship between the spoken word and me. Somehow—like I did with my folks—I had to prove my brother wrong. The opportunity to show my conviction came sooner than expected.

Toward the halfway mark of my senior year with the Genesians, I landed the role of Oscar Madison in Neil Simon's *The Odd Couple*—my first lead role since *Little Shop of Horrors*. During the audition and the first weeks of rehearsals, I perfected a gruff, New York accent that was inspired by one of my favorite actors.

Sporting a catcher's mitt face, an unforgettable Roman nose, a gritty voice, and a vast emotional range, Jack Klugman represented the quintessential everyday man. From comedy to drama, Klugman could effortlessly do it all. During my childhood, I became a great admirer of his distinct nuances. If we weren't catching Jack Klugman solving crimes in *Quincy*, Momma Nettie and I spent our weekend date nights watching Klugman in reruns of *The Odd Couple*, the TV series that was based on Simon's play of the same name.

In the TV version—like in the play—Klugman plays Oscar Madison, a slobbery sportswriter, while Tony Randall portrays Felix Unger, Oscar's anal-retentive best friend. Both divorced and now roommates, Oscar and Felix learn to co-habitat without killing one another in the confines of their New York apartment. Ahead of its time in the late '70s—and a close second to *All In*

The Family as one of the best sitcoms in television history—*The Odd Couple* features Klugman and Randall's unfathomable timing and chemistry, as well as their discipline to not overplay the funny in this smart comedy series.

If I was going to imitate someone, why not imitate the best? On the Genesian stage, I conjured my inner Klugman by mimicking his voice, inflections, and hunched over physicality, as I added girth and age to my performance. But sustaining this quasi-impersonation would only be half the battle.

While keeping my inner Klugman in check, I also had to focus on the technical beats that every Neil Simon play required from its actors. If I missed a word, or if a beat between lines came in too slowly or too quickly, then the funny in the script would land flat. The way Simon wrote, every single word—similar to a musical score—had reason and purpose. Not one bit of dialogue was extraneous, and when executed correctly with rhythmic precision, a certain "Simonian" cadence was created. Rigorously, I tried to adhere to Mr. G.'s decree by staying true with the author's intentions, but even though I carried an accent, this mission was a daunting chore for a stutterer.

At first, Mr. G. seemed to accept the texture I brought to Oscar's voice, nodding from the house without giving me too many notes. This gave me a sense of security, until—a couple of weeks before opening—my director pulled the rug from under me by asking me to use my own voice instead of my pseudo-Klugman. According to Mr. G., the contrived voice didn't suit well with my age. I looked like a boy trying desperately to imitate an older man. It appeared amateurish, almost satirical, which yanked the viewer out of the story.

"Just play the words with your voice, and the character will come out of that," Mr. G. advised.

Mr. G.'s request was like asking a paraplegic to execute a handstand. In a matter of seconds, Mr. G. stripped me of my dependable means, which made me tremble with uncertainty. The life raft was taken away, and I felt like I was dog paddling my way through the play. My brother was right, I didn't have the chops to be an actor.

Days after Mr. G.'s instructions, the rehearsal process took a turn for the worse. I wasn't focused or present. As a result, I started flubbing lines. Instead of worrying about intentions and beats, my concerns turned to whether the next word out of my mouth would be stutter-free. Stopping the flow of the scene, I incessantly asked the stage manager to feed me lines while I was on stage. Sometimes I'd know the line, but hearing the stage manager give me a troubling word was easier to hear and repeat than to say on my own. Out of embarrassment, I relied heavily on paraphrasing and replacement words.

A simple line like, "You want to know what it is, Felix, I'll tell you what it is," would be replaced by me saying, "'Y-You have to know...um...um...wh-what it is...Felix, then I'll um, um say it."

Without the accent, I was nothing on stage, too preoccupied in my own head while I bastardized Simon's classic words. Scott's world eclipsed the safe world I'd built for the past two and a half years on stage. Discombobulated, I kept telling myself that I didn't have a right to be there. Eventually, Mr. G.'s frustration and impatience bubbled to the surface. "That's not what's written, Scott! Stop rewriting the script!"

A part of me resented Mr. G.'s lack of sympathy for my predicament. He was privy to my struggles, so why would he push me into an impossible circumstance? Unable to see the forest through the trees, I allowed my insecurities to control my judgment. In the grand scheme of things, Mr. G. was doing me a favor by ripping my vocal crutches away from me and forcing me to walk on my own. I was just too blind to see it at the time.

Days before opening, Mr. G. disclosed his true motives to me. Stopping the rehearsal in mid-stride, he ordered everyone to take a five as he led me outside of the theater. Under the covered balcony, we went back and forth.

"Look, I can't let you continue in this state," he said. "I'm going to have to put someone else in the role. I'm sorry, but I have to think what's best for the..."

My mouth ran ahead of me as my retort spewed forth, "J-Just let me d-do the damn accent! That's h-how I au-auditioned. That's h-how I r-rehearsed it!"

It was the first time I ever talked back or raised my voice to my mentor. Desperation—not disrespect—took the better part of me. By any means necessary, I would fight for my performance, even if it meant arguing with Mr. G. and at the same time, using someone else's voice on stage.

Rubbing his fingers through his goatee, Mr. G., as usual, didn't say a word at first. I had nothing else to say as well, I had said too much. I held my breath, waiting to hear his response.

"Okay. Use your characterizations," Mr. G. said. But before walking away, he leaned in closer, slipped off his glasses and cleared his throat. "You listen to me now. You are too talented to hide behind something that doesn't bring you...the real YOU to that stage. Until you feel comfortable with who you are, then you'll never be the actor you're meant to be. And you're too talented to let that hinder you."

His words stuck on me as if they were made of Velcro.

A few days later in early November, we opened the play with a sold out audience. Throughout the run, I habitually reflected on Mr. G.'s words. A twinge of guilt stayed with me, reminding me that I was taking the easy way out. Sharpening my dialect and distancing Scott further away from the role was the only way to get by onstage, but I had no more options. That sanctimonious part of me that felt too fragile and too vulnerable to expose had to be locked away in a secret place, concealed from others. Maybe later I could unveil that brittle side of me by saying words in my normal voice, but not at seventeen when all I desperately wanted out of the world was acceptance.

Mr. G.'s prudent lesson was some of the last words he ever imparted to me. *The Odd Couple* would be my last hurrah on the

Genesian stage, and I would never collaborate with Mr. G. again. From then on, I'd see glimpses of him—at graduation and around campus as my senior year drew to a close. The Genesian Players thrived for years to come, even after Mr. G.'s death in 2010. The cancer slowly dimmed the lights on his grand performance, and even his voluminous persona couldn't stop the curtain from lowering. In the course of his forty-year tenure at Archbishop Rummel, Charles Guajardo touched more students than he probably anticipated. In his memory, the Genesian Theater was renamed to The Charles Guajardo Theater. Even though I haven't visited the theater in years, I know Mr. G. is still sitting in the back row, his silhouetted figure leaning forward, critiquing and celebrating every performance, languishing in the tiny empire he had spawned.

"The Thrill Is Gone, Baby"...Never before had BB Kings's signature song reflected my state of mind as I took my closing night bow for *The Odd Couple*. In the blink of an eye, I was stripped of the stage, stripped of my title as an actor, and stripped of the security that came with it. The thrill was definitely gone.

Like any lost soul about to leave the comforts of high school, my certainty in what I wanted to do after graduation remained in limbo. Actually, I knew exactly what I wanted to do, but being the only one with faith in my goal left me doubting. My brother's words still lingered like a rank stench, especially after my last production, where I couldn't even reveal my true self on stage.

Testing the waters, I approached Pop about what I had imagined for myself after graduation. Perhaps he would support me in my acting endeavor. Pop came to most of my plays. He sported a smile when I greeted him after the shows. Why not set the seed in Pop's head about my risky pursuit?

As he sat at the dinner table, Pop grubbed down on a meal that Momma reheated for him. He usually ate alone, since he left his shop so late at night. His dinnertime was the only time he felt relaxed, and I took full advantage of this opportunity. Sitting across from him, I displayed a couple of brochures from Cal Arts and Carnegie Mellon on the table—two prominent conservatories for acting. I'd sent out for them weeks prior, and found the information appealing. I prayed Pop would have the same sentiments.

Before the comment of "I think I want to be an actor," left my mouth, Pop glanced at the brochures, raised his hand and waved it back and forth like he was swatting a fly. "No, goddamit, no! Before you say it, don't!"

The staunchness in his voice shook me, like he was reading my mind. "No more of that actor shit talk. You're gonna get a real degree. Not a shit degree like your brother."

For years, Pop and my brother would clash over his acting major. Momma—playing the peacemaker between the two—coerced Pop into letting my brother attend NYU, only if he earned a scholarship to the university, as well as earning a double major. As Pop put it, "You gotta get something you can fall back on."

Taking Pop's words as gospel, my brother earned a partial scholarship to NYU, and ran to the Big Apple to double major in acting and political science. I, on the other hand, still lacked a scholarship with any reputable acting conservatory. All I had was an acceptance letter from Louisiana State University (LSU) and Loyola University of New Orleans, two colleges that stimulated me as much as getting an enema.

"You ain't gonna end up hungry and poor for the rest of your life," Pop continued to explain to me. "I didn't bust my ass all these years to see my sons screw up. And I won't let it happen." He rubbed his hands together, over the callus scars and cracked fingers that had seen years of manual labor. "I kept quiet about you in those plays, and let you do them. It was good for your stuttering thing, I know that. But now it's time to buckle down and live in the real world. Play time is over."

Pop's blunt remarks were persuasive. My options crashed and burned in a matter of minutes, but I realized I couldn't make it in the real world of theater with a damaged voice and an arsenal of accents. Who was I kidding? I had to face my present circumstance that lay before me, as I tried to block out any remaining desires to be an actor. I had to find something more tangible and dependable in order to assuage my insecurities, and to please Pop, as well as Momma, who would later tell me, "You're the drifter of the family, baby. You're like a gypsy, just floating by. You should listen to Daddy, and just get a degree."

I wasn't fluent enough, audacious enough, or courageous enough to be an actor. In my opinion, I took my final bow after appearing in *The Odd Couple*. The time had come to move on and leave the stage to the professionals.

26 *Trust the Laxatives*

"We should look to the mind, and not to the outward appearance."
—Aesop

A stickler for education, my parent's didn't allow me to skip a semester so that I could "find myself." I had to make a choice, and fast. Deadlines were approaching, and if I waited too long to enroll in college classes, I may be out of a semester— meaning full time at Pop's shop. I didn't want to choose LSU or Loyola, so I dragged my heels until it was too late. My heart lay elsewhere—on some stage in some conservatory in some far off state.

Shortly after, Loyola's deadline for enrollment came and went. With my limited choices, I ventured to Baton Rouge to attend LSU. During my first semester in '91, I declared the first non-art major that came to mind, Criminal Justice. I guess reruns of *Quincy* and *Starsky and Hutch* sparked my interest more than I realized.

Anyone who is left thrashing in their sea of hopelessness usually turns to the most accessible distractions to numb the sorrow. For me, those distractions included drinking and partying. As affluent as LSU preached itself to be, they offered every type of drunken amusement. It was a big country town that valued food, beer, and football. Being dragged away at midnight by dorm neighbors to go honkey-tonking became an ongoing ritual. Not only was chucking back five to ten beers a speedy escape, but when I drank, my stuttering diminished. Perfect speech emanated from me as the stagnate taste of beer and whiskey stained my mouth. In retrospect, liver damage and blacking out were careless and selfish, but back then I thought they were small prices to pay for fluency, especially when I asked a random girl to join me in a two-step without a hitch to my voice. I prayed Momma Nettie wasn't looking down at my late night binges.

As partying evolved into a nightly ritual, I morphed into someone else; an abstract version of me who looked for a fight, and sometimes got one. Willing to entertain him once again, The Hulk came for a visit. Scraps between some faceless drunk and me usually brought my bar nights to a close. I had grown out of control, a far cry from the high school student who abided by a structured schedule. As a result, I skipped classes, my grades slipped, and my weight increased. I gained the infamous "freshman fifteen," or in my case, the "freshman thirty." I gorged in the cafeteria, eating my troublesome thoughts away. Sloth and drunkenness were tools used to drown the potential of who I could become.

It wasn't long before my parents vocalized their concerns about my slipping grades. Pop and his strict Marine discipline threatened that if I didn't clean up my act, he vowed to intervene, which included pulling the plug on my education, any type of housing, and overhead expenditures. The fear of giving up school and having to work in Pop's shop for the rest of my life instantly woke me up from my stupor.

Heeding their warning, I organized my time wisely, cut out all partying and picked up a retail job at JC Penny. For a stutterer, the job was easy to secure and maintain. During the job interview, I kept my responses to "yes, ma'am," and "no, ma'am," as an interviewer rattled off some questions. When I got the job, I made sure I stayed away from the phones by offering my assistance in the storage area. Since the older employees preferred greeting customers and handling orders on the phone, they welcomed my willingness to work in the back. I guess we all benefited from my desperate diversions.

Another outlet that provided rejuvenation to my soul was in a creative writing class—a last minute extra-curriculum class I elected to take. To my delight, I found the written exercises fun and exciting as I organized my thoughts in a creative format.

During one particular class, the professor placed a graded paper on the edge of my desk—a paper I had written about my childhood. In two hours, I regurgitated my memories of Momma Nettie onto the typed, double-spaced pages. The assignment was like second nature to me; it flowed from my hands, and the big A at the top of the page proved my confidence in the assignment. I beamed a satisfied smile that probably caught the attention of a student who sat next to me, an auburn-hair beauty. Like many women on campus, she was out of my league.

"Whoa, how'd you ace that?" she asked me.

Her slight Cajun accent told me she hailed from some rural area in Louisiana. Her name was Melissa and she came from a country community called Franklin, sixty miles east of Baton Rouge. A beauty in a small town, Melissa left the simple life in Franklin and moved to Baton Rouge, where she hoped to continue her modeling career and get her degree. As a side job, she was a personal trainer.

"You seem like you're good at all this writing. I ain't. Could you help a sista out?" Only a girl who needed help in class would talk to a misfit like me, and getting a glimpse of her red D minus on the top of her paper, I could tell she needed all the help she could get.

We agreed to meet once a week at a coffee house that was down the street from campus. During our meetings, I'd glance over her stories, highlight the holes in her plot points, and underline her grammatical errors, which greatly accumulated with each turn of the page. But who was I to judge? I had an overweight figure that needed trimming and a voice that needed work—we all lacked in some area in our lives. Soon, I found myself rewriting her papers. In exchange, she offered her fitness expertise to get me in shape.

As Melissa noted, "I'm gonna work your ass hard, but I promise you'll shed them pounds." Those Franklin girls always had a way with words.

The next few weeks found me huffing and puffing as the muggy air gripped my lungs from our daily jog. Ahead of me, Melissa sprinted like she had jet propellers in her shoes. I stayed focused on her legs and her trim body as I worked to keep up. I had to man up and keep the stride going. Cramps and urges to vomit on the side of the road were a common occurrence, yet I moved forward. I couldn't let Melissa see my weaknesses.

One night, after a strenuous jog through Melissa's neighborhood, I plopped down on a lawn chair in front of her apartment. She came out with two huge glasses of water and a small container of aluminum squares that resembled a gum packet. Melissa pressed on a tiny square and popped out what was concealed in the foil, a soft brown substance that looked like a tiny brownie.

"W-What's that?" I asked.

"Just something to help keep the figure in check," said Melissa as she slid the brown square into her mouth.

Noticing my interest as I peered over to take a closer look, Melissa held up the foiled squares. "You want one?"

Hesitation hit me at first. Nancy Reagan's anti-drug campaign raced through my moral conscience, *Just say no to drugs, Scotty.*

"It's fine," Melissa said with abject confidence. "It ain't gonna kill you. It'll just keep the weight down."

She pushed on the foil and dropped the brown square into my hand. "You're welcome," she said in her cheeky way.

"D-Do I just swallow?" I asked.

"Nope, just chew on the sucka. It tastes okay."

It tasted like old licorice. She handed me the packet and ordered me to take them once a day, either after lunch or an hour before dinner. I should've asked Melissa what it was, but her beauty and charming disposition hazed my common sense. That night I would learn the price for having blind trust.

Around midnight I charged into my dorm bathroom. My stomach grumbled and it felt like my insides were about to burst out. I sat on the toilet for what seemed like forever, moaning in discomfort, and cursing the name of Melissa.

When I called her, she calmly responded, "It's laxatives, darlin.' Nothin' to them. You'll need 'em if you're gonna lose that gut."

27 Animating Rejection

"I really wish I was less of a thinking man and more of a fool not afraid of rejection."
—Billy Joel

Like an illusionist, most stutterers are masters at diverting attention away from our speech impediment to a more positive attribute of ourselves. These manifested diversions come in many forms. As shown in my younger years, silence and a forced smile is a common tool used to hide the deficiency. Sports and other physical affiliations—from the armed forces to martial arts—are careers some stutterers pursue so we are judged more on how we perform than on how we speak. Holding true to the adage, "Beauty is fifty percent illusion," another common ploy involves sculpting and shaping our bodies so that verdicts are based more on how a stutterer appears than on his vocal capability. Vehemently following this latter persuasion, I dedicated months to shedding the pounds through jogging and munching on laxatives. And as a result—like an alluring book cover housing empty pages—I sported a more attractive body that deflected attention away from my broken voice.

After losing thirty pounds, I received remarks that my ears had never experienced. "Wow, Scotty, looking good," to "Geez, you really lost some weight" were just some of the observations that took me by surprise. Additionally, I would get quick, flirtatious glances from random girls as they passed by me. I was by no means Don Juan, but for a guy who wasn't accustomed to smiles and winks from the opposite sex, I was taken aback by how others perceived me in a positive light, especially now that I wasn't on stage any longer.

One day at JC Penny, a younger co-worker cornered me in the storage room, and asked if I wanted to have dinner with her.

Thinking that perhaps she was pulling a practical joke on me, I quickly said no. It was just too good to be true.

Another friend of mine offered to set me up with her roommate, to which I reluctantly agreed. The roommate and I had a lovely dinner, while I let her do most of the talking. This had become my usual modus operandi when going on these new dating excursions. Hiding my stuttering, yet showing off my new physique with tighter shirts and fitted jeans, was the perfect tactic to appear in control and flawless. Finally, I was on my way to being the leading man again.

Like any addiction, my workout regiment took precedence over anything else. I enjoyed the attention, and wanted to make sure the compliments continued. Slowly developing a neurotic tendency, I weighed in four times a day. When I lost two pounds, I wanted to lose two more, then another two. Because of my cravings for physical perfection, the laxative intakes evolved into an everyday occurrence. I'd take them before dinner—just like Melissa prescribed—and then later that night I'd release what I ate in the toilet. Because of the laxatives, I developed intense stomachaches along with heavy heart palpitations, but it was worth the discomfort.

After rushing to the bathroom three times in two hours, I called Melissa and asked her if my frequent bowel movement was a normal bodily reaction. My laxative advisor assured me, "It'll happen here and there. Believe me, you're fine. Your body is just getting used to it." I prayed she was right.

As my obsession grew to attain an immaculate physique, my monotonous lifestyle at LSU became unbearable, and I soon felt too claustrophobic in my surroundings. I didn't fit into the big college lifestyle that had 35,000 students roaming about, and the constant mêlée to find my individuality among the masses grew tiresome. I needed out. I needed to feel like an artist, and fast. I racked my brain, trying to figure out my next move. Unbeknownst to me, my inspiration came that summer in a far off city called Orlando.

Boiling in the Florida humidity, I handed out ice cream bars to parched tourists who resembled panting hyenas looking for a drop of water. My polyester uniform had no ventilation. The sweat stung my eyes as it dripped down my brow. But through my discomfort, I still carried a cheerful disposition, for I was serving frozen treats at the happiest place on earth, Walt Disney World.

Through the Walt Disney College Program, college students from around the world were carefully selected to work minimum-wage jobs for a summer in Orlando. In exchange, we were housed in apartments, attended business courses, accumulated school credit, toured various facilities in the park, and had an opportunity to get our foot into the door of the monolithic corporation. For the interview — which took place at LSU through their outreach program — all I had to do was put on a cheesy "Disney" smile, respond with small answers, and fill out an application as well as complete an essay titled "How Has Disney Affected My Life?" Like auditions, interviews were becoming easier to master, especially when it came to written procedures. Hence, in the summer of '92 as I just finished my first year at LSU, I was hired to work in Disney's food and beverage department.

Flipping burgers, taking out the trash while fireworks blasted above me, and selling dry iced fruit bars were my obligations during those dog days of summer. According to my nineteen-year-old sentiments, I just landed the most coveted job in the history of employment; I was part of something bigger, something so far away from the imprisonment of home and the dullness of LSU.

My new responsibilities for Disney were the least intimidating when it came to my stuttering. "Y-You want to g-go that way," followed by a "H-Have a n-nice day," were the usual responses I uttered to guests who asked for directions. But who cared if I sounded like Woody Woodpecker? Everyone was there to have a good time, and they never gave my stammering responses a second thought. The elation I felt from the job made me less self-conscious.

Because drawing and sketching were a big part of my upbringing, I jumped at the chance to take an in-depth tour of Disney's animation facilities. Almost five years prior to my employment, Disney animation had a resurge in popularity with the arrival of *Little Mermaid* in 1988. Since then, the studio capitalized on their near-moratorium art form with the release of *Aladdin*, and *Beauty and The Beast*. With their forthcoming films, *Pocahontas* and *Mulan*, Disney was reaching new heights with their stapled animation. But behind the cells and the lovable characters that illuminated on the screen, the real celebrities who breathed life into the celluloid sat in their fancy bungalows located in the back lot of Disney's MGM Studios.

Two things gripped my interest during the tour of the animation department: Animators were actors behind a pencil, and animators were treated like movie stars because of the unique talent they brought to a high-demand brand of storytelling. Their prominence was evident in their BMWs and Jaguars adorning the parking lot, the catered food that graced the lobby, and their own 24-hour private gym and basketball courts. It was like a fraternity house for the eccentrics.

When I walked into the corridors, The Rolling Stones filtered from the overhead speakers, and there was a carefree banter between the artists. Toys and action figures hung from the rafters or balanced on the sides of their desks—the same action figures I had in my room many years ago. A charming cockiness exuded from the animators, who acted more like the lost boys of Neverland than architects of a burgeoning new industry. At one time, they were misfits who probably never got the girl, or were the last to be chosen in a dodge ball game. Now they were the rock stars of the lot.

Peeking into random offices, I watched animators etch mind-boggling sequences on their huge inclined desks. Observing their hands and arms whip about was like watching a maestro orchestrate his music, but instead of a tuba or violin, the animator had his imagination and blue pencil at his beck and call. As I watched them demonstrate their artistry, a familiar euphoric sensation pulsated through me, similar to when I said my first line on the Genesian stage. *You can do this*, I repeated to myself as the tour came to a close.

Not only did the whole scenario charm me and re-stimulate my inner artist, but it also helped devise another plan in my head. As an animator I could impress my family, embody the wealthy son who drove the sports car, and attach my last name—our family's name— to classic films. No more did I have to trip on words to perform; now I could be a star with pencil and paper. The romance, glitz and glamour of animation seduced me more than anything else.

After the college program, I made it a priority to build up an illustration portfolio, so I could apply to various art colleges. Reverting back to my sketching days, I dedicated my time to drawing and honing in on my talents. Hours upon hours were spent hovering over sheets of paper as I shaded and meticulously detailed every picture. It wasn't long until schoolwork and class hours became more of annoyance than a responsibility. To compensate for my impatience in escaping the drivel lifestyle that LSU offered, I ramped up my workouts—jogging eight miles instead of six, taking more laxatives, and attaining the outer perfection that gave me an identity.

"You wanna be a friggin' clown?"

That was Pop's initial response when I told him I wanted to attend Ringling School of Art and Design, one of the most predominate art schools that had an intensive animation department.

I tried to explain. "P-Pop, it's n-not a circus school, it's one of the b-best art schools th-that D-Disney selects from for their animators."

To concentrate more on what I had to convey, Pop turned off the lawnmower and slipped his hands into his pockets. The scent of newly cut grass pinched my nose as my father and I stood on the front lawn.

"So let me get this straight," Pop said, "you're gonna be drawing cartoons for a living now? Is that a way to make money?"

"Y-Yeah. B-But now they make a lot of m-money. L-Like six figures a year." Pop's face turned from concern to confusion. The whole animation idea still wasn't sticking well with him. I had to press the facts further if I was going to make any headway. Composing my thoughts and making sure I didn't get ahead of myself, I told Pop about the art school—how John Ringling of Ringling, Barnum & Bailey Circus fame opened a museum and an art school in Sarasota, Florida, how the school grew into the most recognized art school for leading animators and graphic artists, and how Ringling had accepted me into their illustration/animation department with a partial scholarship, as well as accepting most of my common curriculum classes from LSU.

After I finished my informal presentation, Pop sighed, looked up and said, "If this is how you wanna waste your life, then go ahead, but just get a degree."

I vowed that I would, noting that Ringling offered a bachelor in fine arts once I graduated. If only for a little while, this satisfied Pop's unceasing demand for me to have a backup plan. Soon after, Momma somewhat went along with my choice. "If this is what you really want..."

As I prepared to move to Sarasota, an unmentionable skepticism still lingered in the back of my head. Could it have been the acting bug still biting me? Even if I felt the sting, I shook off the pangs and stuck with the sketching because it was my only golden ticket out of LSU, and my last chance to feel uncommon. Besides, telling my parents in the spring of '93 that I wanted to be an actor was more taboo than any time prior. The reason for my trepidation to impart anything about acting was linked to my brother, and his sudden misfortunes in New York.

Eating Ramen noodles from morning to night, running from audition to audition with no encouraging outcome, and living in an apartment that resembled a Russian gulag, my brother called it quits. After eight months in New York as an actor, my brother moved on, noting that acting wasn't for him. He landed a job at a national television station in Washington, D.C., and started a career in journalism. I guess his political science degree came into better use than he had previously expected.

Even though my brother explained, "I just got burned out on the acting, that's why I left," I knew better. It was the rejection—having someone tell him that he wasn't good enough, or good looking enough, or talented enough—that compelled my brother to move on from actor to reporter. I could deeply relate to his rejections.

My parents used my brother's sudden career change as a prime example to their theorem that actors either quit or collect unemployment. So I kept a lid on the acting pursuit by suppressing any aspirations that still remained. Even though I was about to turn twenty, I still wanted to please, and still valued my worth to what others thought of me, especially from my parents. I longed to satisfy them and to have them believe that I wasn't a stuttering handicap, that I was fully capable to be on my own, and that I was Able instead of Cain. My parents' happiness and acceptance still dictated my actions. That in itself was a recipe for disaster.

28 Round Trip Meal

"Do I want to die from the inside out or the outside in?"
—Laurie Halse Anderson, Wintergirls

The Sarasota sun pelted down on me as I dashed onto the school campus. My daily six-mile sprint had been arduous that particular day. But staying true to what Melissa taught me, I kept the run at a healthy pace, not giving up, and not giving in as I pushed my leg muscles to the brink of fatigue. Dehydration and lack of food was getting the best of me. Dinner from last night ended up in the toilet, and I skipped breakfast that morning. I was famished, but I had grown accustomed to that familiar feeling.

Running onto campus, I looked down at my watch. I had twenty minutes to spare before figure drawing class. I raced to the cafeteria and ordered two full servings of Chinese noodles with chicken and beef. I scarfed down both plates within five minutes. It was about time I listened to my body. My tummy craved food, and after filling it, the body shakes dissipated.

Thirty minutes later, as I sat in my figure drawing class, a gush of panic overwhelmed me. I couldn't concentrate on my half-finished sketch of the naked model in front of me. All I could think about were the two giant portions of food digesting in my gut and turning into fat. I dropped my pencil, bolted out of class, and found the nearest bathroom.

Inside, I washed my hands, took strands of tissue, and ran into the nearest stall. I flushed the toilet twice, bent down, and placed my two fingers on the back of my tongue. The noodles and bits of meat burst out of my mouth. I cleaned my hands, rinsed my mouth, popped a piece of gum and returned to class.

The art of the round trip meal took less than one minute. Since starting Ringling, I developed an acquired compulsion to stick my finger down my throat in order to sustain my slim figure. I'd graduated from the laxatives, and entered the dark realm of an eating disorder. The stomach burns, lethargy, and the sting in my throat were an acquired feeling. But even if it hurt, I blocked it out. No way was I going to let my parents see me as the fat kid again, or the tubby stuttering son who didn't know what the hell he was doing in life. I had to play the part to a tee. I kept the illusion going, even though my internal misery permeated.

Bulimia was a symptom to the truth I longed to suppress, and that truth kept gnawing at me. From the moment I entered Ringling's campus and took my first illustration class, a sudden doubt covered over me. Like a groom second-guessing his vows at the altar, I knew I had made the wrong decision. Sure, I chose to be part of an artistic environment that exceeded LSU, and the sketching and drawings I produced brought a temporary accomplishment, but a void still remained—an unsaid void that still whispered to me, telling me to leave in an instant. *Be the actor*, it kept saying.

Even if I wanted to leave, I'd have to face the grand jury. Pop would say, "I told you so," and I would prove Momma's theory that I was the gypsy of the family. Thus, another son would be labeled a quitter.

But as much as I tried to delude myself with sketches, I missed the words—the spoken words. At night, when my bunkmate was sound asleep, I clicked on my flashlight and delved into the plays I had long neglected. With Williams, O'Neil, and Chekov in my hands, I had a late night date with the greats in my upper bunk as I whispered their well-structured dialogue. Yet during the day, I felt the suppressing shackles. The more I felt the inner struggles and shunned any desires to be an actor, the more I stuck the finger down my throat and made way to a more emaciated version of me. In due time, I withered away to one hundred and thirty-five pounds. According to my contorted sense of appearance, this seemed healthy for a 5' 11" guy, until objective, honest voices woke me from my delusional perspective.

The anticipation was too much to take. Several months had passed since I last saw them, but now I was minutes away from meeting up with Pop and Momma at Disney World, just an hour and a half north of Ringling. I couldn't wait for them to see the improved me—the trimmed, slim, lean Scott. Their faces would beam with joy at my achievement. All I had to do was smile and perform the role.

I knocked on their hotel door. Momma answered. With a big grin on my face, my arms extended out. Momma's face changed from elation to horror in a matter of seconds. Turning away, she covered her face, and screamed, "No! No!"

I asked her what was wrong, but all she could do was sit on the edge of the bed and weep into her hands. Pop exited the bathroom with a newspaper in one hand and a towel in the other. He looked at me in the same fashion as Momma.

"My boy," Momma cried out through her covered hands. "My boy is sick."

Noting Momma's reaction, I looked to my left and glared at my abnormal reflection in the mirror. My collarbone protruded from under my shirt. My face was drawn in; hallowed circles surrounded my eyes. Acne covered my cheeks, forehead, and chin. My medium button up shirt draped on my frail frame like a bed sheet over a tall lamp. For the first time, I took notice of the emaciated monster before me.

Momma woke me from my epiphany when I heard her cry out, "My boy has AIDS!"

Pop grabbed me by the arm, pushed me outside and shut the door behind us. "Are you sick?"

"No, sir."

"You look sick, son. Your Momma thinks you have AIDS. Do you?"

"No, P-P-Pop. I p-promise. It's…something else."

"What's going on? Tell me. Man to man, tell me the truth."

The truth…the goddamn truth? I thought, staring at a pleading version of Pop. Prior to two minutes ago, every time I saw myself in the mirror I thought I was looking at a fat guy, a flawed guy, and a guy with a Frankenstein tongue who spoke like something out of a horror movie. Since I could remember, I concentrated more on my imperfections than on my attributes, so I tried to override these negative feelings by feebly achieving perfection. I focused more on the rejections and the repulsions because it was easier; because I didn't want the responsibility to live the life I knew I was meant to live.

Pop gripped my arms and said, "Whatever is going on, you need to take care of this, or I will!"

I leaned on Pop, and wept like a baby. Pop hugged me tightly, his hands pressing on my back. "Son, your ribs," he whispered. "Jesus Christ, I can feel your ribs. Please, please let us help you."

I clutched onto Pop as parts of his shirt crumpled under my hands. I held on to him for dear life outside of that hotel room.

"What, son. What is it?"

As my face buried in Pop's shoulder, I told him, "I-I just want you to b-be proud of me."

He hugged me tightly, like he had never done before. "Son, I've always been proud of you."

I rejoiced in hearing this with open arms. The vulnerability between us was palpable, so I felt compelled to continue on. "This p-place isn't for me. I'm sorry, b-but I want to b-be an actor. That's w-what I'm meant to d-do." It's amazing when you are stripped of every disguise, every tactic, and there are no more hiding places to burrow under. That is when the truth is easier to convey.

By Pop's body going rigid, I could tell he wasn't ready to hear it, but it was the truth. For the first time in a long time, I spoke my truth out loud, without contemplating the outcome.

My tears turned from sorrow to relief, as tranquility washed over me.

Since my classes were already paid in full, I agreed to continue my courses with Ringling until the end of the second semester. Additionally, I promised to take care of my eating disorder by studying nutrition, sticking to a healthy eating plan, and committing myself to a more conducive workout regiment. For some unexplained reason, my parents believed me, and had faith that I would find a solution—in my own way. I guess they already assumed I would be resistant in seeking psychiatric help.

Like an inmate anticipating his release date, I felt an inner peace knowing my time at the art school was coming to an end. During that time I re-evaluated my relationship with food, and strategized my next plan of attack once I left Ringling. Whatever course I chose, I knew I couldn't let the fear of my voice and the fear of my family's opinion dictate my future any longer. Whatever detrimental guises I had acquired along the way had to come to an end. And the only way to silence the pestering demons was to pursue what I was born to do. Weeks before the end of my second semester at Ringling, a promising prospect presented itself; and for the first time in three years, I had a chance to perform in front of a live audience once again.

29 Staying Gold

"We fear discovering that we are more than we think we are. More than our parents/ children /teachers think we are. We fear that we actually possess the talent that our still, small voice tells us."
—Steven Pressfield

Two years older than I, Tony represented the classic Renaissance man. Bordering on neuroticism, he could paint, write, act, and direct with an unprecedented intensity. He was the quintessential perfectionist. Before long, Tony's appetite for theater and the performing arts made its way onto Ringling's campus. His one goal before graduating was to produce and direct a play starring Ringling students and its faculty members. Thus in the spring of 1994, Tony would put his passions to good use in the production of *The Outsiders*—a play based on the popular 1982 Francis Ford Coppola movie and the book of the same name. With Tony's invitation to audition, I leaped at the opportunity to be in another play.

Auditioning for *The Outsiders* brought me back to my days at the Genesians where I crafted a foolproof audition technique. Because I watched the film many times on HBO and studied the book in my high school junior lit class, the feel of the story and the Oklahoman accent that *The Outsiders* required was easy to summon. The audition was inspiring and uplifting—both best friends for any stutterer who hadn't performed in quite a while. Rehearsing my lines for the audition while supporting a thick Midwestern draw, I relished in the words, as it quenched my craving to be on stage again. The day after I auditioned, Tony informed me that I was cast in the pivotal role of Johnny Cade, a role I connected with in a profound way.

In the play, the seventeen-year old Johnny Cade suffers from an abusive home, and the only acceptance in his abandoned world comes from a local gang called the Greasers. With these outcasts, Johnny finds love, a brotherly adoption, and a calling to stick up for those who are helpless, which ultimately leads to his demise. I knew the texture of Johnny even before we began rehearsals. Similar to Johnny's life, I found acceptance and loyalty with misfits who were like me—outside of the norm and alike in my reclusiveness. During the rehearsals, I would recall my relationship with Pauley many times.

The more I rehearsed the play—which would debut and close on the last weekend of our semester—the less I desired to stick my finger in the back of my mouth. I finally responded to the silent whisper in my head that had preached to me for so long. In return, I experienced an unparalleled self-assurance on and offstage. The longing to be a perfect specimen slowly diminished.

In the Ringling cafeteria-turned-pseudo-theater, I could feel the Saturday night audience as they sat in their silence. Off in the wings, I waited to enter the stage and recite my final monologue at the end of the show. I had gone the distance in the last two hours, performing in a stutter-free accent that had intention and commitment behind it. Closing my eyes and envisioning Johnny, I prepared to tackle the most challenging monologue ever to come out of my mouth. In the monologue, Johnny—who has passed away after saving children in a burning church—narrates a letter that he has written to his best friend, Ponyboy.

Making my entrance while sporting a leather jacket and rolled up jeans, the spotlight shot its beam down on me. I peered out into the audience, and said my final lines, " 'I've been thinking about it, and that poem, that guy that wrote it, he meant you are gold when you're a kid, like green. When you're a kid everything is new, dawn. It's just...when you get used to everything, it's day. Like the way you dig sunsets, Pony. That's Gold. Keep it that way, it's a good way to be.' "

Silhouetted heads faced me. Staring back at them, I heeded Johnny's words as I recalled the memory of my uninhibited imagination from childhood, the same imagination that helped me deal with my stuttering and the complications that accompanied it. Like Johnny said, I had to return to that childlike simplicity to do the impossible—to be on stage and to speak the written word. *Just let go,* I silently told myself.

My mouth quivered as I said my last line, a line that Momma Nettie would have probably said to me on her deathbed, "Stay gold, Pony, stay gold." Nothing else existed in my present circumstance. I wasn't just Scott personifying Johnny anymore; I was someone else beyond the script, beyond my imperfect voice.

As the lights dimmed and the foreboding strum of a guitar played in the background, bringing the play to an end, I heard slight sniffles from the crowd. The stage went black. In the darkness, I ran off stage. Emotionally disoriented, I didn't know where I was, or who was around me. I bumped into Tony, who uttered warm congratulations to me. But I couldn't retain everything he had to say. My head was somewhere else, still involved in the scene, still wrapped up in the intensity of it all. Suddenly, I heard one clap, then a few more from the audience, and then a multitude of claps ensued as I made my way to the dressing room. I didn't realize it at the time but I had skipped my curtain call.

Shutting the dressing room door behind me, I awoke from my fuzziness and wept, not as Johnny, but as Scott, a guy who without a doubt knew what he was meant to do. The confidence, acceptance, and victory I felt on stage could not be ignored, and never again could it be discounted. This is where I belonged. I wanted more of it, but to earn it in the long run, I had to throw my whole being into the pursuit.

Later, while calming my overwhelming emotions in the solitude of the locked dressing room, I looked around and noticed sketches and paintings hanging on the walls. Former to present students had donated their various theses to the school cafeteria—all were framed in perfection. As I sat there half naked, I realized I could never paint, draw, or shade like these masters. My heart wasn't in it. My heart lay somewhere else. What I did on the stage just five minutes ago, that was my perfection, my mastery.

The morning after the closing of the play, I taped a note on Tony's dorm door, thanking him for the opportunity. On the bottom of the note, I wrote down my address, phone number, and a reminder to "keep in touch."

I bolted to my car, revved up the engine, and careened down the highway. I looked in my rearview mirror. Even though luggage and boxed items in my back seat blocked my view, I didn't need to see what was behind me. I was not going back. Hours later, I approached a sign that read: "INTERSTATE 10 WEST: THIS EXIT."

I weaved onto the exit westward bound. The sun was setting in front of me. I took off my sunglasses and allowed my face to bask in the radiant shine. I knew where I was going. I knew where I was headed. I knew what I wanted to do with my life. *Stay gold, Scotty, stay gold.*

30 Iambic Pentameters

"God has given you one face, and you make yourself another."
—*William Shakespeare*

There's freedom and clarity that comes when we repel the forces that tell us we're not good enough or talented enough to attain our dreams. Ironically, we author these resistant forces and adhere to them as if they were gospel. But once we revolt against these self-manifested lies and start down the road that may lead us to our destiny, ideas and plans are created that are clear, concrete, and forever weaved into our perseverance.

The forty pounds I had gained comforted my parents, and assured them that I was on the verge of a healthier me. With a firm voice, I announced my future plans to my parents, who listened attentively from across the booth in the crowded Chinese restaurant. My proposal to them was clear and to the point, where most of the responsibility lay heavily upon my shoulders. For starters, I would be attending Loyola University of New Orleans and majoring in English Writing and Literature. While taking classes and living at home to save money, I'd wait tables on the side, immerse myself in the New Orleans theater community, and keep my GPA at a 3.4 or higher. Once I graduated and earned enough money, I'd move to either New York or Los Angeles to pursue an acting career.

During the summers, I'd continue my employment at Disney World. Since two summers prior, I had advanced from food and beverages to an area that was more suitable to my talents, the entertainment division. From strapping on an intricate puppet based on one of the characters from *The Lion*

King, to prancing around in a furry outfit for the Main Street parade, my job was far from glamorous, but it wasn't half bad.

After vocalizing my two and a half year commitment, my parents took a moment to process my plans. Pessimistic about my move to a big city upon graduation, Momma was cautious. "It ain't easy out there, Scotty." She reminded me of my brother's difficult start in New York, and she was correct in her assessment.

But I was resolute. "F-fooling myself is not easy, either." Nervously brushing the palms of my hands on the table, I continued, "Ya'll are g-going to have to r-realize, I'm not him."

By this time, my brother had a propitious career as an on-air TV journalist for a major religious channel. Acting was far behind him, yet he used his acting chops to tell the news and give a dramatic flare to his on-screen persona.

Pop butted in. "Your brother is getting paid good now. Once he gave up that stupid acting shit..." The broken record never stopped skipping.

Breaking the tension, the waiter arrived at the table and slid my chicken and mushroom in front of me. Taking my chopsticks, I picked at the tender meat and devoured the meal within a matter of five minutes. Not another word came from me. It wasn't worth it. Audibly convincing my folks was a waste of breath. I'd have to show them.

A rigorous schedule awaited me when I started Loyola—a private university established by the Jesuits and named after the order's founder, Ignatius Loyola. In the heart of The Garden District, the one hundred-year-old university is still nestled on St. Charles Avenue where the magnolia trees flourish and streetcars screech by. Entering the campus and experiencing the poetic nostalgia that only The Garden District has to offer, one can't help but feel like they are in the middle of a Tennessee Williams play. But for me, I had no time to consider the campus' romantic side. My motivation and newfound goals reminded me that I had things to do, and a limited time to do it.

Since graduating from Rummel, my stay at Loyola was the most focused I had ever been. Writing and immersing myself in literature, I felt like Loyola was a better fit for me, far more than my previous schools. Adding on to my eight-hour day courses, and my waiter job three nights a week at the local Applebee's, I decided to dive into theater once again.

Loyola's theater department had three theaters on campus—a large commercial theater for the theater department, a more elegant theater for operas and special events, and a black box—an experimental theater for undergrad productions. Within these theaters, Loyola produced close to eight to ten shows a year, and they opened their casting to all members of the student body. Longing to keep my skills sharp, I took full advantage of the open calls, and auditioned for the first show of that season, an old chestnut of a play called *Stage Door*. The play—written in the '30s—focuses on a group of young and aspiring actresses in a New York City boardinghouse, and a successful producer who falls madly in love with one of the actresses.

Copying the tonality of Cary Grant with a touch of Alex Trebeck, I conjured up an accent and posture that fit the highfalutin, well-spoken producer, Alex Powell. Besides mastering the accent, I made it a top priority to learn my audition sides verbatim for the audition; familiarity with Powell's lines, texture, and rhythm led to no stuttering. Unlike many of my high school auditions, I greeted the five-member production team with my own voice as I walked into Loyola's two-hundred seat theater, and, in costume, proceeded to do the scene off book, committed to the dialect and my rehearsed blocking.

A week later, I booked the role, reshuffled my schedule to accommodate rehearsals, and pissed off a handful of theater majors. Since I was on their turf, some of the theater majors felt they deserved first dibs to the meatier roles, and not some English major.

Many Loyola productions followed in the next two years, which I had the great honor to appear in—*Antigone, Three Penny Opera, Frankenstein, Romeo and Juliet, Henry IV,* and *All in the Timing.* They were an eclectic collection of plays with skilled directors at the helm, and I had the privilege to perform each role with accents and distinct postures. My trick of the trade to conceal my stuttering on stage had proven resourceful, and the directors agreed, which meant they never ordered me to stop my artificial, yet fitting, voices. But this ruse would only last for so long as I entered another chapter in my life that would challenge my true voice.

She weighed only one hundred pounds soaking wet. Her dyed jet-black hair swooped down, hiding any remaining wrinkles that her facelift couldn't stretch out. She embodied the desire to sustain the last remnants of her youth. Never in my wildest dreams did I predict that this high-maintenance woman named Franny would change the course of my life.

A director and instructor in Loyola's theater department, the fifty-two-year-old Franny never let her vanities affect her classroom. She was the consummate professional and an insightful teacher. For an acting professor, she ran a tight ship, and always asked for the truth from her actors. Often auditing her classes and agreeing with her sensible approach to classical acting, I learned much from Franny about how to approach a role, how to break down every line of dialogue, and how to treat the classics as if they were contemporary pieces.

"Shakespeare's words aren't foreign if you know what he's saying. It's your job to convey the meaning," Franny would always preach.

From the moment we met, Franny and I jelled well together. Her remarks to my diction were full of praise. Once, she asked if I followed the Alexander technique—founded by the great Australian actor, F.M. Alexander. His technique alleviates tension in breathing and vocal capacity by relaxation, proper posture, and an acute awareness on stage. Unaware of this technique at the time, I lied to Franny and told her that I did adhere to Alexander's method. A part of my Catholic consciousness wished I didn't have to lie, but if I was carrying out the ruse for Franny and everyone else on campus, why not commit to it a hundred percent?

One night at a closing night party for *Romeo and Juliet* at The Contemporary Arts Center in downtown New Orleans, Franny cornered me and said, "Your diction on stage is remarkable. You, my boy, have an acquired technique. Just don't tell any of the other students I said that, love. There are some jealous bitches among us, you understand, don't you?" I have no idea whether Franny was just stroking my ego, but I bought into her compliment at the time. Sometimes we believe what we want to hear.

The performance that Franny referred to was my portrayal of the mischievous and spiteful Mercutio, Romeo's comrade. Perhaps what caught Franny's attention was the playfulness, the athleticism, and the flirtatious nature the director asked me to bring to the role. Or perhaps it was my Standard English dialect and diction I'd copied from my brother, meshed with a touch of Laurence Olivier. Franny assumed I studied some intricate technique for my performance, but all I did was imitate, recreate, and listen. Somehow, I glided stealthily under her radar.

In my defense, because I found Shakespeare's iambic pentameter easy to perform, I did have more of an unrestrained and sprightly feel on stage when I recited The Bard's words. With the five hard beats throughout a typical stanza—da, DUM, da, DUM, da, DUM, da, DUM, da, DUM—I felt as if I was singing a song. Even though I still depended on a dialect as a crutch, musical beats and lyrical rhythms in the sixteenth century dialogue lent some comfort to my uncertain speech pattern.

As the courtyard party buzzed around us, Franny grabbed my arm and pulled me to the side. By her hard grip and her tightened brow slightly rising, I could tell she had something significant to share with me.

"How would you feel about acting abroad...taking acting courses in England for the summer?" My ears perked. I stared at Franny's collagen lips, trying to detect if perhaps she was bamboozling me.

"R-Really?" I asked. Franny didn't pick up on my stuttering all that much. Most of the director's didn't.

"If you want to, I can get you in without an audition." Franny affirmed. "I teach courses there every summer. It's a classical intensive, and I think you would do really well. Are you interested?"

Almost sixteen years later, I'm still thankful I agreed to Franny's offer.

31 A Midsummer Night's Lesson

"To cultivate an English accent is already a departure away from what you are."
—Sean Connery

Loyal to her word, Franny found a way to get me into the prestigious summer program without an audition, and without going through rigorous callbacks in New York and Los Angeles. I still had to fork over the $3,700 to attend—which I barely had at my disposal—but ultimately I found the means. Under the wire, I made the summer tuition by working at Pop's shop, performing for a month at Disney, and taking extra shifts at Applebee's.

For a stutterer who waited tables, I found the job to be less arduous than I had previously predicted. Instead of saying "Can I help you?" when greeting a table—which included the devilish bad no-no "C" at the front of the sentence—I relied more on replacement letters like "W" at the beginning of my alternative greeting, as well as the soft "H" and the easy "S," as in, "Welcome, how may I be of service?" Even though another bad no-no like "B" was at the center of the phrase, it didn't hinder me in the least. As long as I got through the first two words, I was home free.

Upon finishing my rehearsed greeting, I would let the customers rattle off their orders, and add a bright smile into the mix. It was amazing how grinning, listening, and serving people without saying that much helped me earn higher tips. As I learned from being around actors, listening and letting others speak was a strategy that worked to my advantage.

After laboring like a workhorse for the next four months, I soon found myself surrounded by fifty international actors who made up that summer's British American Drama Academy's (BADA)

Midsummer in Oxford Program, an annual six-week intensive held at Baliol College in Oxford University. Established by Julliard—and in conjunction with The University of California—BADA's purpose was to reach out beyond the shores of England to actors from around the world who wanted formal and intensive training in classical theater with some of the top British actors and directors.

From the moment I entered the elegant historical walls of Oxford—where classes were held and where I'd reside—an indescribable familiarity coursed through me, and I felt right at home. I had previously pictured similar surroundings where Sir Conan Doyle's stories and my imagination danced with one another. The Tudor homes and cobblestone sidewalks reminded me of Doyle's infamous sleuth who ran about solving crimes—even though Oxford was seventy miles away from Sherlock's London.

Soon my amorous sentiments subsided when the grueling courses went into full swing. Depending on the student's experience, talent, and expertise, the classes at the academy were broken up into three categories: Intermediate, Advanced, and Professional. For some reason Franny signed me into the Professional Class, which was made up of sixteen highly-trained actors. The professional title may have been a bit ostentatious to some, but we had to prove our "professional" worth in more ways than one.

Ten hours of movement class, vocal exercises, fight training, Shakespearean acting, and Jacobean text studies encompassed our early mornings to late evenings. Having BADA's Director of Program and the dean of Julliard, Michael Khan, criticize our prepared scenes added wrinkles to my face and a couple white hairs to my head. Rehearsing scenes and dissecting heavy Elizabethan and Jacobean lingo until three in the morning didn't help alleviate any pressures, either. The mixture of work overload and jet lag weighed heavily upon me to the point where my brain was full and my body was in much need of a good Rip Van Winkle slumber. With the lack of sleep came the strain to my voice and the slight stuttering hiccups in my scenes, even when my voice was cloaked behind a dialect.

Clearly, I was in way over my head, and I began to second-guess my choice in attending the summer intensive. Lying to Franny about my supposed knowledge of the Alexander technique probably came at a hefty price. But as I pressed on—and to my relief—I did excel in a couple of classes, movement and stage combat. It was easier for me to show off my athleticism more so than my voice, which included wielding rapiers, stretching my body for strikes, taking dramatic hits, and manipulating my body to resemble some zoo animal.

Ironically, another valuable course I found gratifying was the voice class. Our voice instructor Carolyn was a patient and boisterous Irish woman who hailed from The Royal Academy of Dramatic Arts. Even though she believed in the natural way of things by going braless and deodorant-less, Carolyn reminded me of Hambuga's protocols, like putting a cork in between my teeth while I enunciated words, breathing through the nose and out the mouth when feeling flustered on stage, finding support in the diaphragm, connecting consonants by elongating vowels, and where to properly breathe in Shakespearean text. One lesson she fervently concentrated on was emphasizing verbs in the dialogue. As Carolyn explained, "You must put the stress on the verb of the sentence. The listener, whether he knows it or not, will be more attentive when hearing the verb. The lines become more active in the audience's mind."

Her assorted lessons helped me more as a stutterer than as an actor. I learned how to relax in the text, and how to connect emotions to the classical words by breathing at the correct places in the dialogue. I would put her exercises to good use for the better part of my career.

Some of the international actors in my class included a famous MTV reality celebrity from Ireland, a Scottish actor who appeared in popular action movies, a New Zealander who had been a famous teenager actress in her homeland, and a striking Australian sitcom actress named Raven. To say Raven was my school crush would've been an understatement, as she soon became more of an obsession. Her spiked highlighted hair and her puckish demeanor added to her beauty. On and offstage, she had an ease about her, which made her the class favorite. Innately having the vivacity of a twelve-year old, Raven held an uncanny enthusiasm when engaging someone. She embraced everyone, held him or her intensely, always asking, "How are you, dear?" Her attentiveness was never disingenuous; on the contrary, the most disengaging and aloof person would instantly open up to her warmth. Everyone was drawn to her quirkiness, including me.

Staring at her constantly from afar and being seduced by her enigmatic yet alluring presence onstage became a normal episode for me. In some way I wanted to connect with this petite spark plug, preferably onstage in a scripted scene where I knew the outcome, and where I felt somewhat in control.

After the first two weeks of classes, I began to get into the swing of things. I had grown accustomed to my instructors' critiques, and soon I welcomed their sharp criticisms. I didn't want to be coddled anymore. I was determined to learn as much as I could. Similar to Mr. G.'s style—an aggressive and candid style I learned to appreciate—I wanted to be beaten down so the instructors could build me back up. Sure, my mindset had a masochistic twist to it, yet to be the best I had to hear the good news along with the bad news and, subsequently, learn from both. But throughout this classical boot camp, there was one habit I couldn't relinquish. The accents. I'd clung onto them like a child holding onto his safety blanket.

In class, my now perfected Shakespearean accent kept my secret concealed onstage, while my social drinking offstage made me fluent and stutter-free at the local pubs with fellow classmates. Nearing the halfway point of our summer intensives, I thought I would go undetected as a stutterer. But without warning, my infatuation with Raven and my guarded speech impediment collided and, inevitably, I was exposed.

As a director, Ian was as sharp and meticulous as they came. Always sporting his signature blue slack, blue Polo shirt, navy blue sweater tied around the shoulders, short white hair, and pursed lips, this Artistic Director of the Glasgow Theater carried his eccentricities and opinions in an unruly and charismatic manner, like every Welshman. Over a drink or two, Ian shared his opinions with me, which included the following:

"*Braveheart* was full of bullocks, it didn't happen that way. Men in skirts never won that easily."

"The most underrated actor in the theater is Pete Postlethwaite, hands down!"

"The American theater is turning into a McDonald's drive thru, where the masses want a quick fix instead of a play with substance."

Ian's candor when engaging an actor—or anyone, for that matter—was full of zeal and intensity. He never let an artificial moment pass by onstage, even though he still hadn't responded to my phony accent. But all that would change.

During Ian's class, an actor made a spastic flicker of the arm while performing a soliloquy, which forced Ian to inquire, "Excuse me, but was that?"

By the blank expression on the actor, I could tell Ian's interruption jolted the young student.

Ian uncrossed his legs in the front row of the small theater and explained, "Your fidgety movements on stage are getting in the way of the text. Don't do that. Be strong. Be still. Let us hear the words instead of being distracted by needless movements."

Hunched over in the second row, I waited for my turn to arrive, which followed the twitchy actor. Any minute, I would ascend the small stage and deliver my Edgar speech from *King Lear* with a Scottish brogue. For a week I had worked on the soliloquy, and I was certain my punctuation, diction, and accent would bring satisfaction not only to Ian, but to Raven as well, who sat a row behind me.

Before I knew it, Ian shouted from over his shoulder, "Scott, let's see what you've got!" Standing, I reached down and picked up my pages of dialogue from the ground. Behind me, I heard a cheeky Australian voice, "Go get 'em, cowboy."

I looked up. Raven's distinguishable spiked blonde hair and grooved dimples faced me. She winked. I smiled back. *I'm going to ace this.*

"Let's go, Scott," shouted Ian, "before Christ comes back a second time."

Taking my place center stage, I cleared my throat and said the first stanza with my Scottish brogue that would make Sean Connery smile with pride, "Thou nature art my goddess, to thy services I am abound. Wherefore..."

Before I could continue on, Ian stopped me dead in my tracks. "Excuse me but what is this accent you're giving me?" he asked.

Looking down, I could see Ian leaning forward, his index finger pressed against his puckered lips. My eyes scanned the theater, trying to organize my thoughts and come up with an excuse. "Because I would sound like a broken motor if I didn't use an accent," was what I really wanted to tell my instructor. Sixteen blank faces stared up at me from the theater as Ian prodded me further, "You've been using these renaissance fair accents throughout the course, and I must stop you now."

The jig was up. In front of the entire class, I had been called out. Suddenly, my attention turned to Raven in the third row. A pen dangled from her mouth, fluttering up and down between her teeth. *Be careful. Don't embarrass yourself, Scott. Not in front of her!* My thoughts turned to Mr. G.'s words from almost eight years prior, telling me I had to be comfortable with myself onstage and offstage if I was to reflect any sort of truth in my performances.

Ian stood and placed both his hands onto the stage, leaning on them as if he may do a couple of push-ups. His blue eyes pierced up at me. "You don't need an accent when performing Shakespeare. Why do American actors always think they have to sound like bloody Mr. Belvedere when performing classics? God gave you your own voice, use it!"

After a few guffaws from the class, I nodded to let Ian know I understood, but I had no clue of what to do next.

"Good, take it from the top," Ian instructed me. "And this time, let's hear your *own* voice."

I couldn't catch my breath. My throat tightened. Without the accent, I knew what would probably transpire if I opened my mouth.

I couldn't stutter in front of my Australian goddess, or in front of my highly influential instructor. As I looked down at the verse in my hands, I convinced myself I didn't have a right to be on the stage, that I was way over my head. *You're a phony. Run!*

"C-C-Can I have a moment?" I asked Ian.

"Of course. We'll listen to another soliloquy," said Ian as he pointed to his left. "You, Raven, are you ready?"

"Yep, Capt'n" replied the Australian as she stood up from her chair.

Before Raven made her way onto the stage, I was already out the door. The nearest pub was within a two-block radius outside of campus, close enough for a sip of courage. After my third pint, I had all intentions to return to the theater and use my slight inebriation to my advantage. But as I ordered my fifth Guinness, the bar spun around me. Performing while drunk was an area I still had to perfect, and I was by no means Richard Burton. I decided to remain at the bar for another hour, at least until I sobered up. I was safe for now, quiet for now — the calm before the storm.

32 The Voice of Pain

"Acting is a matter of giving away secrets."
—Ellen Barkin

Two nights after my shameful moment in Ian's class, I gulped back a lager as our school-sponsored party raged in the distance. Drinking had once again become an everyday occurrence to stabilize my voice and the insecurities that tagged alongside it. The party was an outdoor affair, and since the unpredictable English humidity had me sweating like a mule on the dance floor, I needed some fresh air.

Sitting on the bank of the river, I took in my enchanted surroundings. The flowers gave off a floral scent that intoxicated me more than the lager bubbling in my gullet. Resembling dragonflies gliding on the river, punters floated back and forth. Just then, above the rap music that bumped and thumped from the party, I heard feet pressing down on grass just behind me. The careful footsteps came closer. I didn't turn around. If I did, I would have probably fallen over from the alcohol swirling through my head.

"You never came back to class the other day," Raven said as she squatted next to me, referring to my speedy exit out of Ian's class.

With the liquid courage supporting my stuttering, I said, "Oh, yeah, well, I had a date with a girl at the Turf Tavern." I was feeling a little saucy, and I thought I'd play with my school crush for a bit.

Showing some interest in my story, Raven moved in closer, "A date...with whom?"

"Okay, I'll tell you, but you can't tell anyone." In a low tone, I said, "Her first name is Guin. And her last name is Ness."

Mouthing the name, Raven caught on. On cue, she leaned back and laughed. I didn't think it was that funny, but clearly she did.

Maybe she was more intoxicated than I thought, or maybe my delivery was sharper when I was smashed.

Placing her hand on my lap, she said, "You're a cheeky bugger, aren't you?" I winked back. If this was flirting, we were both doing a damn good job.

She leaned over and grabbed the beer from my hand. She took a swig. The suds made a small mustache on her upper lip. "Next time you bail on a class, take me. Maybe we can get smashed together."

I let out a drunken chuckle as the butterflies banged around in my stomach. I may have been inebriated, but I sure as hell knew when a saucy Australian was coming on to me.

Later, in the wee hours of dawn, I found myself under Raven's spell as we shared kisses on her bed. When the morning light peaked through her bedroom window, I was suddenly carried away by the awe-inspiring view. Like snapping a Polaroid, I wanted to freeze-frame the sun's rays kissing the chimneys and slanted roofs. The purple and orange hues reflected something out of a Monet painting.

"I like it here," Raven whispered as she rested her head onto my chest. "It's such a nice break from the crap I have to put up with."

I propped up on my elbow, and brushed the hair from her eyes. "Wh-Wh-What crap?" I asked. The stutter came back as the alcohol wore off, but I didn't think too much of it.

She sat up and wrapped her arms around her knees. "Agents, and press events, and being the next best thing. I have a crazy life back in Sydney."

Wish I had that life, I thought to myself.

Raven grunted in annoyance. "I don't know how to deal with it. I forget who I am sometimes. That's why I'm here...to get back to basics." She reached out for my hand. "Why are you here, silly boy?"

I wasn't sure if she was asking why I was attending the school, or why I was lying in her single size bed as our bodies began to interlace with one another. Whatever her implications, I didn't answer her question. All I did was lean in and passionately kiss her. I had no intention of telling her the truth, of how I came to jolly ole' England to prove to myself that I wasn't a freak; that a skilled, successful actor resided behind my damaged voice. I just had to find it, even if it was across the Atlantic.

But this midsummer morning was not the time to talk of such things. I wanted to give Raven her fantasy. I wanted her to forget her reality, and I longed to forget mine in the process. In that moment, I was perfection—her sturdy white knight. I had rehearsed the role many times before.

As the weeks progressed, so did Raven's sudden disinterest in me. She never waved back or made eye contact with me after our night of escape. When we passed each other in the quad, she looked the other way. Slowly, I started feeling like a used commodity, a quick fix that Raven chewed on and then spit to the side. I was a pit stop in her erratic, rollercoaster life, yet I was the one who put myself in that position. It was a role I could perform but never sustain. My heart wasn't designed to become such a luxury for others, not anymore.

Sooner than I thought, my present frustrations escalated when Ian announced that I would be performing the Edgar soliloquy in the next Thursday class, but this time I was instructed to use my voice. To silence my apprehensions, I hit the booze harder than before.

One night, after a few shots of an English concoction, I pounded on Raven's door. Romance and alcohol owned me that night, obviously a bad combination. When Raven answered her door, she held a copy of *Coriolanus* in one hand and her reading glasses in the other. Trying to bring some humor to our awkward moment, she told me she was doing a little light reading. She chuckled. I didn't. I got to the point.

"Why do you keep ignoring me?" I asked in my drunken, stutter-free voice.

She leaned on the opened door and took in a sigh. I longed for that connection, that spark in her gaze that she used to give me in class. "You're a great fella, and I think we moved too fast. But we're leaving the school soon, and I don't want to get attached. Look, you don't know me, and I don't know you, so let's not get ahead of ourselves. You understand, don't you, silly boy?"

Silly boy. Those two words were worse than a smack across the face. But what stung the most was that I knew she was right. How foolish to think that some Aussie goddess could make all my pain go away, or that I could reciprocate the feeling as well. What did I expect from her? That she was the blue fairy to my Pinocchio? With one touch of her magic wand she could make me into a real stutter-free boy? The time had come to take on my responsibilities and to stop hiding, stop latching onto the next easy fix, stop my undying search for someone or something to save me. Women, bulimia, booze, art school, and accents—they were all synonymous; they were theatrical stages I had created to become this fantastical leading man for everyone, except for myself; the perfect detours from pursuing my life-long task. As I left Raven standing in her doorway, I knew what I had to do, and it would be one of the hardest undertakings I had ever performed.

On that early Thursday morning before everyone was awake, I sat in the solitude of the tranquil Baliol quad. I couldn't sleep. The anticipation was too much to bear. In four hours I'd perform the soliloquy without the accent, and without the artificial me. Sure, I could get hammered at 7 A.M. and let the booze guide me through a stutter-free performance, but the running had to stop. Sooner or later I'd have to step up and confront the bully inside of me. He was stronger than Johnny Finger. He was more spiteful than my brother's abusive words. This inner bully had power, hissing his lies that every stutterer hears; "You're going to fail. No one is going to like you. Just be quiet."

In class, I kept my head tucked, staring at the floor and preparing myself for the unforeseeable outcome. "You're next Scott," Ian said. Complying, I made my way to the stage. Raven sat in the middle row. I couldn't look at her as I took center stage.

"Remember, Mr. Damian, no accent," Ian ordered. "Now, whenever you're ready."

Taking a full deep, diaphragm breath, I saw the first word in my head. "Thou." Placing my tongue between my teeth, I tried to push it out in my own register. Spit sputtered out of my mouth. I heard a couple of people fidget in their seats, uncomfortable at the sight before them as my head shook back and forth. Inhaling again and trying to control my gyrations, I gave it another whirl. The same disastrous result occurred again as my face contorted.

My first inclination was to make a run for it, jump into a taxi, head to Heathrow Airport, and fly back home. But if I ran now, I'd never return. I'd always be running. Out of the corner of my eye, I caught Raven looking up at me. We locked eyes, and my mind shifted. I wasn't on stage any longer. The faces looking at me from the audience slowly dissipated from my periphery. The sight of Raven ignited a reaction as my thoughts voyaged somewhere else. An all-encompassing determination set in, yet the determination wasn't to win Raven's affections. This resolve was deeper than her or any type of need to be loved or praised.

Beginning the monologue again, my mouth ran ahead of me. I had no more room for doubts or reservations. My purpose took over and became my rowboat on a gale of recollections as I recited my lines with no airs and no dialects:

"Thou, Nature, art my goddess; to thy law

My services are bound."

Performing Carolyn's lesson of breathing where the text permitted, I took in another deep breath. The stuttering was nowhere to be found. I forged on.

"Wherefore should I

Stand in the plague of custom, and permit

The curiosity of nations to deprive me,

For that I am some twelve or fourteen moonshines

Lag of a brother? Why bastard? Wherefore base?"

Breathe, I reminded myself. My heavy, tingling breath carried gravitas with it as the air filled my lungs and landed on the thin surface of my soul. Each word from the soliloquy resonated in my core, reflecting everything I wanted to say to those who doubted my voice, and to the bully who had twisted and turned inside of me since I was a child. The soliloquy was to all of those cynical entities. No one was innocent in this courtroom. I leaned in, keeping my gaze on Raven—the involuntary muse of this scene.

"When my dimensions are as well compact,
My mind as generous, and my shape as true,
As honest madam's issue? Why brand they us
With base? With baseness? Bastardy? Base, base?"
I took in another breath.

"Who, in the lusty stealth of nature, take
More composition and fierce quality
Than doth, within a dull, stale, tired bed,
Go to th' creating a whole tribe of fops
Got 'tween asleep and wake?"

With every punch of consonants and every extension of vowels, I grew closer to the actor I was meant to be, connecting the words of the Bard to my own life. Franny was right. It was my responsibility to convey Shakespeare's words, and in the process, I granted myself the right to speak from the heart in my own God-given voice.

"I grow; I prosper.
Now, gods, stand up for bastards!"

Lowering my head, I was done. A silence waked over the small theater. For a moment, I forgot my bearings. Soon, I woke from my dramatic possession by the applause ringing throughout the theater. Glancing down at the front row, I caught site of Ian participating in the applause. "Well, done, boyo! Well done," Ian remarked as he made his way to the edge of the stage.

He spread his arms along the rim of the high stage. "My God, where did all that come from?" asked Ian in what seemed like a rhetorical question.

I answered anyway. "Pain."

33 The Oddest of Couples

"Comedy is simply a funny way of being serious."
—Peter Ustinov

One of the perks while attending BADA was having celebrity instructors speak to us and share their wisdom about the industry. Alan Rickman, Fiona Shaw, Uta Hagen, and Derek Jacobi were just a few of the notable personalities who popped in and out of our classes, imparting their sentiments about how it was to be an artist and not just a "familiar face" on screen. But out of all them, there was one celebrity who stuck out above the rest, and who I was determined to meet face-to-face.

Standing before us inside the crowded meeting hall, he spoke to the students with fervor. Still sporting a lanky, lean figure, the then seventy-six-year-old Tony Randall spoke passionately of acting as his arms gestured like violent pinwheels. A youthful elegance permeated from his voice. I still saw hints of Felix Unger in him, even though he wore a more saggy face and grayer hair since his sitcom days. His passion about acting was contagious as he talked about the depths of his process. His sixty years of theater expertise was evident in the advice he imparted to us.

"To do!" Tony Randall exclaimed. "Acting is doing. You enter the stage, you do. You leave the stage, you do! The stage is a place of constant doing. You don't say things. You do things on stage. Even when speaking, you're doing to gain something!"

As Tony Randall's lecture came to an end, various students surrounded the veteran actor like ants to sugar, but I didn't participate. I had other plans in mind. Stepping outside into the Oxford quad, I waited for Tony to exit. I wanted to create an opportune moment to speak to him without the congestion and interruption of photos or autographs. Sitting on a bench just below a hovering tree, I whispered to myself, rehearsing the words I would convey to him.

With his entourage in tow, Tony exited the hall and into the quad. He made his way toward the entrance of the campus. Immediately, I tried to catch up with him, hoping we could have a moment to ourselves.

"Mr. Randall?" I blurted out. When his red, tired eyes met mine, I froze. Without a TV screen between us, Tony seemed so available and personal. Because of my irrepressible excitement, my mouth and throat stiffened from the surreal situation before me. My eyes fluttered back, pushing to get the first word out.

Sensing I was having a hard time speaking, Tony put his hand on my forearm, and with the most sympathetic gaze, he asked, "Are you alright, young man?"

His touch soothed me, and broke me out of my blockage. "S-Sorry, I g-got excited..." I took in a deeper breath, slowed my heart rate and said, "I'm a b-big fan. I kn-now every episode of *The Odd Couple* by heart."

"God, I hope I was good," he said.

I laughed. He chuckled. "Th-Thank you for all you've d-done. You and J-Jack K-Klugman really left an impression on me."

With honest gratitude, Tony thanked me and then said, "If you're not too busy this summer with classes, you should come see Jack and I do *The Odd Couple* on stage in London. We'll be there 'til the end of August."

I perked up. "You...and Jack K-Klugman?"

"Yes, the one in the same. At least I hope it's him. Or maybe I've been performing with someone else." He released another slight snicker.

As the image of Klugman dashed through my thoughts, Tony Randall patted my shoulder again. "Young man, what is your name?"

"Scott."

"Well, Scott, when you come see the play, stick around after and ask the porter to let you up. Come say hi, will you? I look forward to seeing you then."

And with that momentous invite, Tony headed toward the exit of the campus. All I could do was stare at Tony shuffling away, until he morphed into a tiny speck of a human. My weekend getaway to London couldn't come any faster.

I needed a break, and going to see two familiar faces that I had grown to love was the perfect remedy. I had triumphantly performed in Ian's class by using my own voice, but campus life and the pressures of studies were getting a little monotonous and overbearing—two sworn enemies for any artist. Plus, the sight of Raven every day still gnawed at me.

That Saturday, I hopped on a morning bus to London in order catch a matinee performance of *The Odd Couple*. Arriving in London, I entered the West End Theater, which felt more like an oven than an old English playhouse—no air conditioning, and it was the middle of a scorching summer. I squirmed in my seat, impatiently waiting to see Felix and Oscar live and in person. *Eat your heart out Momma Nettie*, I thought as the curtain rose.

The lights came up, and I held my breath when Jack Klugman entered the stage with his baseball hat turned backwards, while a stogie protruded out of the corner of his mouth. When Klugman said his first line, I mouthed the line in unison. Even though I did the Genesian production almost six years prior, I still knew the lines verbatim—great dialogue is never forgotten.

As the play continued, my sentiments soon faded, and I felt as if something was off kilter. My attention turned from the dialogue to how Klugman delivered his lines. His voice sounded harsher, raspier, like he had a bad case of laryngitis. He'd lost something; no more did he have that manly resonating voice that came with his infamous under bite. He sounded injured, tired, and almost delicate.

Next to me, an elderly, Cockney woman whispered to herself, "Too bad. Just awful."

I leaned over to her. Maybe she was thinking what I was thinking. I whispered, "Wh-What's wr-wrong with him?"

She paused for a second as her finger pointed to Klugman on stage, "He had throat cancer. They took part of his vocal cord. Dreadful."

I slid my hands along the arm of the chair. I fidgeted. My shoe anxiously tapped on the floor. My heart sank as I averted my eyes away from the stage—I guess my emotions got the better part of me. Until I grew accustomed to his frail voice toward the end of the first act, I couldn't look at Klugman. It was heart-wrenching to witness, not because I was disgusted. On the contrary, I felt intense empathy for the veteran actor. I knew how it was to have a voice that was imperfect, holding you back from delivering so much. As others around him spoke loudly and eloquently on stage, Jack was stuck in a battle with his voice. Though his inflections were limited and he had a hoarse drone to his voice, Klugman still earned the laughs and had the "Simonian" rhythm down to a science. The actor gave his all in that matinee performance.

After the show, I heaved up the steep staircase. Just moments prior, the porter called up to the dressing room and told "Mr. Randall" that I had arrived. Tony ordered the porter to let me up to the third floor in the back of the theater. Nearing the dressing room, I was tickled pink that Felix Unger had just requested me to come upstairs for a visit.

With no presumptions of what to expect, I knocked on the dressing room door with a star in the center of it. Tony opened it. Quickly, I darted my attention away from him, trying not to bust out laughing at the sight before me. There was Tony Randall in the doorway, wearing a tie and buttoned shirt, caked on make-up, tissue flaring from his collar, no trousers, only boxers, knee-high socks, and a brown iced concoction in his left hand.

"Hello, Scott. Did you like the show?" Tony greeted me, nonchalantly ignoring his present situation.

His question didn't register at first. Noting my reluctant response, Tony apologized, "Oh, yes, sorry for my appearance. It's stifling hot. No air conditioning. Please forgive me. We have an evening performance…must cool off."

Like a muffled foghorn, Jack yelled out from the other room, "Tony…Tony? Do you want the turkey sandwich or the ham sandwich?"

Tony turned his face to the side, "I'm at the door, Jack. I'm with a guest."

I stared in wonderment at the whole scenario. An episode of *The Odd Couple* was unfolding right in front of me, and I felt as if I was cast as their sitcom neighbor, asking to borrow a pinch of sugar.

Jack poked his head from the other room. "Everything okay, Tony?"

"I'm fine. Come and meet one of the students from BADA."

With a limp to his walk, Klugman crossed over to the entranceway while chomping on a half eaten sandwich. His face looked older. His eyelids draped. His makeup was thickly applied, but it couldn't hide the wearisome wrinkles on his face. But behind the caked makeup, I still saw remnants of Quincy.

"Who's this?" Klugman asked in a voice that sounded like he had shattered glass stuck in the back of his throat.

Tony introduced us, "Scott, Jack, Jack, Scott." Klugman shook my hand hard and tight. His hold was unforgettable.

"N-nice t-t-to meet you, Mr. Klugman." The excitement got the best of my voice.

"Call me, Jack." Klugman said. "Well, gotta go rest the voice." Jack pointed to his lower neck. "Two shows today, you know? Nice to meet you, young man."

Wobbling back, Klugman disappeared into the void of the massive dressing room. So badly I wanted to explain how much I idolized him, how his unique voice guided me through the perilous waters of an almost certain stuttering performance, and how a redheaded spitfire once had a crush on him. But I didn't want to pester Klugman with such sentiments. My stay was long enough.

Tony shook my hand, and thanked me for stopping by—his gracious and polite manners always intact. I returned the thanks and made my way down the stairs, past the porter, and onto the busy street of the West End. I stopped, took a breather on the corner, and digested the whole experience. Here were two veteran actors entering the twilight of their careers. They embodied older versions of themselves, yet they continued on, hoping to go out with a bang, hoping to continue their legacy to the finish, with no bitterness attached to their soon-to-be final curtain call.

How many times did someone tell Tony Randall that he was just too damn old to perform in live theater? How many doctors told Jack Klugman that he could never act again, that his voice was gone, and that it would never come back? Yet these thespian soldiers ventured on, ignoring the consensus and the ignorant assumptions that probably inundated them to no end. They may have moved more slowly, but they were fastidious in their determination, still acting, and still doing what they loved to do.

On the busy corner, watching taxis and buses zoom past me, I prayed to God that one day, when I reached the twilight of my years, I would still be running the marathon beyond my expectations, and beyond the fear of my voice. Like Randall and Klugman, I would never live my life in accordance to others' perceptions. Tony Randall was right, like life, in order to act, you have to do. Do. Do. Do, no matter what.

34 Band of Heathens

"Some people bring out the worst in you, others bring out the best, and then there are those remarkably rare, addictive ones who just bring out the most. Of everything. They make you feel so alive that you'd follow them straight into hell, just to keep getting your fix."
—Kren Marie Moning, Shadowfever

The confidence that BADA instilled in me gave me the courage to pack up, move out, and make my way to Los Angeles once I graduated. My parents thought it was just a phase; they believed the gypsy would return home, just like he did before. Momma said I could always come back if things didn't pan out, no questions asked. Like a bookie, Pop had his own predictions on the matter, which he would've doubled down if I made a bet with him. He believed I'd be back in six months, and he did anything in his power to sabotage my plans.

"You know you have to be good looking to make it in the movies," Pop said as I shoved my bags into the trunk of my Camry.

In Pop's practical world, he wanted me to stay, get a master's degree, maybe a Ph.D in something I had no desire in pursuing. But my folks had no clue of the resolve pounding inside of me. Like before, the more disparagement I heard from them, the more I wanted to prove them wrong. I was leaving, running away from their pedestrian life. Oxford proved I had a voice, my own voice, and it needed to be heard.

Los Angeles wasn't paved in gold, and that bitch wasn't going to give me anything for free. I had to work hard, to the point of exhaustion if I was going to be heard. Finding a place to live in LaLa-land didn't come easily either. For weeks I slept on my friend's couch while he and his unemployed roommate clomped by me in the wee hours of the morning, grubbing on cold pizza after their late night partying. The apartment reeked of rotten pizza and sweaty feet, but I couldn't complain. I was a paid guest in their house, shelling out two hundred dollars a month to use a musky couch as a temporary bed. All I could do was suck it up, find a job, and save enough money to get an apartment of my own.

Instead of landing a job serving at a restaurant or organizing letters in some studio mailroom—like most actors who move to L.A.—fate had me performing in the most random of places, Knott's Berry Farm's Wild West Stunt Show. Labeled as the first theme park in America, Knott's Berry Farm was founded by Walter Knott, the jelly and jam giant of Southern California who was known locally for his Chicken Dinner Restaurant. Attracting a horde of hungry visitors in the late '40s, Knott erected an Old West town adjacent to the restaurant to entertain his hungry customers while they waited hours for available tables. Soon, Knott's Wild West facades grew into a popular theme park, only to be overshadowed by the opening of another theme park right down the road called Disneyland.

Auditioning for the stunt show proved less threatening than my previous auditions. I read a few lines for Knott's creative team with an accent that would've given Matthew McConaughey a run for his money. After executing forward rolls and some punches, Knott's entertainment division asked me to join their show. Gratefully, I accepted. In return, I got to fulfill most men's fantasies—I was a cowboy, baby!

Wearing a black Stetson, riding boots and strapping on a gun holster, I cracked whips, perfected my fast draw, and tumbled thirty feet off buildings with some of the best guys I ever encountered. Most of the men who made up our twenty-member stunt team were a band of misfits—my kind of dudes. There was Bubba, the ex-linebacker for the Eagles who wrecked his knee, ended his career as a football player, and moved from Minnesota to pursue another risky career in show business as a stuntman. Eddie was the Iowan correctional officer turned actor and writer whose stocky muscle-bound frame, sharp gaze and pointy jowl exuded toughness, yet he'd

get misty-eyed over a kid in a wheelchair. There was the good ol'
Southern boy named Rich, who painted like Rembrandt, and
catapulted a flip that made professional wrestlers cringe. Aaron was
the real-estate rep turned cinematographer who worked Knott's just
for shits and giggles because, as he explained it, "I love being a
cowboy." There was Cola, a marital artist who fought for his identity
as a Jamaican/Caucasian and felt the sting of racism at an early age.
Matt was the handsome one, and the only true singer on the team,
who could hold a high C note longer than he could hold his arch
when performing a 40-foot fall.

We were full of contradictions and alike in angst, yet we were a
band of heathens who all had a dream, a common goal—to sustain a
successful career in Hollyweird while having fun in the process. We
were poor as church mice, but we had the time of our lives playing
Doc Holliday and getting paid for it. Like a frat house, our stunt team
participated in mischievous antics—water balloon fights, fake shoot
outs, and throwing cold buckets of water on a victim who happened
to be taking a hot shower. The testosterone was palpable, and I
leaped into the rough housing with no remorse. The boys bestowed a
nickname upon me—Rooster—and I lived up to the name. I crowed
with a belting caw at a moment's notice, and made sure I was the
biggest chicken in the coup. The first one to jump naked in the pool at
a raging party, or haze a newbie on our stunt team, I held onto the
title of Rooster with the utmost commitment. Adding onto my
reputation, I'd make out with any girl who found a Sicilian-looking
cowboy remotely attractive, and telling the boys of my overnight
revelries was even more fulfilling. Subconsciously, I was still adding
layer upon layer to my leading man exteriors, trying to distance
myself further away from the stuttering boy who still resided within
me.

As our team developed a tighter bond, we soon discovered that
besides our ass-grabbing and rough housing, there were more
common interests between us than we realized. In the late 1990's,
digital filmmaking was beginning to make a huge impact in the
studio system. With a wave of successful, low-budget films, like *The*

Blair Witch Project, and *El Mariachi*, many no-name filmmakers were taking chances with new affordable technology and venturing out to make their own films. During our breaks between stunt shows, the boys and I studied these selected films in our tiny break room. Huddled masses of men congregated around a twenty-four inch TV, pointing out plot points and camera angles. Soon, the poignant question rose among us, "Why can't we make our own movies?"

After brainstorming sessions, our team put Aaron's XL-1 to good use—the first handheld professional digital camera of its kind. Writing shorts and planning shots, we filmed in guerrilla-style fashion. Overnight, or on our days off, we shot in the most random of places—desolate wooded areas, inside cars, or in the hallways of Knott's Radisson hotel at 2 A.M. If one of us wasn't performing in front of the camera, the rest would slide behind the camera, directing, holding a boom mike, or adjusting lights. There were no egos, and no room for divas. We worked efficiently and creatively to capture the best story we could produce for no budget at all. Under the banner of our newly formed company, Branded Maverick Entertainment, we produced and shot an array of genres that reflected our passion for filmmaking.

While on set for one of our comedy capers, titled, *Role of a Lifetime*, another monumental achievement happened to me. It was a simple shot, nothing complicated in the setup. Portraying the lookout out man for a group of actors who moonlit by night as diamond thieves, I had to cross from the hotel elevator and make my way down the hallway to my designated mark. I was to recite three lines into an earpiece as Aaron led the way with his camera pointing towards me. Usually my mind would race with apprehension, like what if I fumble a word? When I get to my mark, will I screw up a line with a bad no-no? Yet, from out of nowhere, and as unpredictable as winning the lottery, the dialogue eased out of me in my own voice, without an accent, trepidation, or self-doubt. The comfort of having a group of guys who felt more like equals rather than a hierarchy brought stability to my voice. In my own way, I was reliving my days with Pauley, and the excitement we shared in telling a story. In that narrow hotel hallway, I let myself enjoy the process as I worried less about the end result. I didn't care if I made a mistake or flubbed a line on set. For a moment, the weight of perfection lifted from my shoulders. I gave myself room to play. What had transpired in Ian's class wasn't a fluke after all.

Stutterers never wake up one morning and—like getting over a cold—the impediment is completely gone. It is a slow, melodic process that comes with time, patience, and certitude. That monumental day of articulation may never happen, but if it does—as in my case—it sneaks up and occurs without the stutterer noticing at first. Like a swimmer who stops to marvel at the miles he's swum, so do stutterers when we pause and reflect on our gradual victory. My time of reflection occurred in the most casual of circumstances, yet the outcome was far from normal.

The conversation wasn't mind altering; it was a routine exchange. Behind the rickety stage of our stunt show, the guys and I convened over a long table, wearing latex gloves to clean our guns. A half-hour before our shift ended, we routinely scrubbed our issued guns, always keeping our babies cleaned and oiled after a long day of shooting blanks. We all had names for our guns. "Betty," "Grim," "Dolly." Buffing and polishing my gun "Scarlet," I discussed our shooting schedule for one of the scenes we were planning on covering the following day.

"So before we film the outdoor scene, we're going to shoot at Aaron's house and film the party scene instead, right?" I asked Eddie as we sprayed our guns with WD-40.

Questions and ideas about our shot list flipped back and forth between us for fifteen minutes. Rich and Eddie would give their opinion. I'd give mine. Suddenly, the whole scenario hit me like a cannonball. Sensing an unexplained emotional response about to explode inside of me, I forced a smile, quietly excused myself from the table, and hurried to our outdoor stage. Like strips of dialogue, I replayed the conversation in my head. The bad no-no's were there in my said words—P's, B's, I's, A's, D's—yet I didn't stammer, or replace hard words with easier words. No gut wrenching hesitation and no buffers were evident, either. For fifteen minutes I had complete elocution with Rich and Eddie. *Was this a fluke? And have I been doing this for some time now?* I asked myself as I tried to recall my most recent conversations. Fully aware that I would probably flub words in future circumstances, I knew that I hadn't vanquished stuttering all together. My nerves would probably grapple with my voice, or my need for perfection would get the best of me. But I'd take it head on, day-by-day, and word-by-word.

For now, I celebrated in the joy of my present victory. At twenty-six years old, I stopped treading water in the high-sea of fluency. Instead, I looked back and acknowledged my accomplishment. I had finally reached articulation in my real world exchanges. Flopping down on a hay barrel, I quietly wept for joy.

35 A Stutterer's Forgiveness

"When you're in a hole, stop digging."
—Denis Healey

As a steady income flowed in from Knott's, I finally had the means to move into my own apartment and invest in my career. Attending actor's workshops, hiring a photographer to take my resume pictures—which sometimes cost more than the photographer's camera—and submitting those said pictures to agents, I took the initiative to find theatrical representation. But trying to sign with an agent in Los Angeles was like finding an In-N-Out in the Serengeti—impossible. Agents wanted name, accredited actors. They didn't want to take a chance with just anyone. Up front, agents wouldn't tell such truths to actors; instead, their excuses ranged from, "We are not taking new clients at this time," to "You have to be in the union before we can consider signing you."

Doors kept shutting, but I wasn't going back home with my tail between my legs, and I sure as hell wasn't going to follow in my brother's footsteps. One thing stuttering taught me was how not to succumb to rejection. So I kept pushing on, looking for a better angle.

In L.A., one way to be seen by industry folk is to showcase yourself in live theater. The antithesis of New York theater, L.A. theater is an almost unprofitable entity for actors and writers alike— except for the occasional charlatan theater owner who charges an exorbitant rental fee. Because of a special 99-seat theater agreement with Actor's Equity, union actors in Los Angeles are allowed to perform in smaller venues---with 99 seats or less---without pay, union breaks, and union benefits. In return, actors are able to perfect their craft, and invite directors, producers, and casting directors to their performances. In New York, it's about the work. In L.A., it's about being seen.

Highly recommended by a fellow Knott's performer, I auditioned for a reputable theater company in Hollywood called Actors Co-op. Located in the Hollywood Presbyterian Church campus—right in the heart of Hollywood—the award-winning Actors Co-op reflected its name to a tee; a non-profit co-op made up of sixty actors whose purpose was to produce six mainstream plays and musicals per season based on their subscribers' interests. Proud to be the only profitable Christian theater company in Los Angeles, Co-op consistently sold out shows in their two 99-seat theaters. But not everyone in L.A. embraced the merging of art and faith; across town, Co-op was labeled "The Holier Than Thou Theater Company."

At first, I carried the same sentiments; the whole scenario seemed too hokey, too safe and too religious for edgy theater. But beyond their Christian ideals in a town riddled with bad, pretentious theater, Actors Co-op had a viable reputation for being one of the most polished and well-organized theater companies in L.A. Plus, after speaking with a few members, and watching a couple of Co-op productions, I concluded that this unique brand of theater brought a New York mindset to Los Angeles. For most Co-op members, doing the work was top priority; being seen by industry people was just an added commodity. Even though I yearned to sign with an agent, the work mentality that Co-op represented resonated with me, so I auditioned for my first L.A. theater company.

To be chosen as a member of Co-op, I faced a slew of interviews as well as an audition process where I had to perform two diverse monologues—one contemporary and one classical. For my audition, I selected a trusty monologue from *The Odd Couple*, and the Edgar soliloquy from *King Lear*. To be sure I aced the audition, I applied my well-rehearsed accents to the words. I didn't want to concern myself with stuttering in front of a bunch of strangers, especially strangers I wanted to impress.

Weeks later, the company accepted me into their award-winning group, and after a while, I discovered what the word "co-op" really meant—selling refreshments during intermission, taking down sets on Monday nights, and ushering for shows on weekends. Like the Genesians, no one was above the tedious labor, and that made me feel right at home. As I watched talented actors perform during my ushering duties, the urge to be on a real stage came gushing back. A sentimental feeling set in, and it reassured me that I had made the right choice in joining the company. But my newfound assurance wouldn't last for too long.

During our Monday night Co-op meetings, where we discussed business matters and came together as a company, time was allotted to pair up into small groups and pray. Interlocking hands with people I hardly knew and praying with them unnerved me. I longed to say lines, not to pray with a bunch of actors I hardly knew. Instantly, I wanted to bow out, tell them thanks, but no thanks to their wanna-be tent revivals.

Being Catholic, I was taught to keep my prayers solemn, and closed off from others—never raising hands, screeching "Alleluia," or reciting scripture with a Billy Graham conviction. As a kid, I prayed to a crucifix that hung above my bed. Just God, St. Dymphna, and I, and a round of requests that one day I would speak in a normal voice. Rosaries and Novenas were commonplace in my household as well, but that was as close to group prayers as I got. Sure, my family would say the occasional mealtime blessing over our dinners, but who didn't in a Catholic home? For my family, Church and faith were private matters, never to be exposed or flaunted about like a new pair of shoes. The only thing that was remotely similar to reciting Scripture in our house was Pop testifying, "Without God, a man has nothing." Praying aloud, speaking in tongues, and being well versed in Scripture was for the Protestants, not the Catholics.

For some odd reason, as the weeks pressed on, an insatiable feeling had me returning to the Co-op meetings. Ironically, I missed the unexplainable peace I felt when I left the meetings. From afar, I'd witness how prayer affected others and the mighty grace that circulated through the meetings for those who had real problems. Drugs, alcoholism, infidelity, porn, and a slew of other vices were discussed during the prayer time, but so was the forgiveness. If I was attracted to edgy material in a script, I was even more engrossed in the edgy reality that crisscrossed in front of me during those Monday night meetings.

After a few meetings, my initial apprehension and intimidation toward the Co-op turned into a sudden surrender. As I gave in and participated more with the group prayers, that same low, gnawing, relentless voice pestered me to no end, but this time it kept whispering, *Forgive*. The word haunted me for days.

A month in as a member of Co-op, I clutched hands with a woman of sixty who'd just lost a loved one in a car accident. She was a character actress who had that recognizable face, but you couldn't pinpoint her name as you snapped your fingers and asked, "Haven't I seen you in something before?"

Bracing to hear her prayer request of grief and loss, I was shocked when she turned to me and gently said, "If you don't mind me being forward, but God told me that you must forgive."

My palms turned sweaty. A chill pulsated up my body. *Who is this voodoo doctor?* I quietly thought. She continued, "I'd like to pray about that, do you mind?" Here was a woman who experienced a traumatic event, yet she wanted to pray for me. My initial response was to deny her on-target assessment, but I bowed my head and listened to her soft prayer. As the woman's voice penetrated my soul, a revelation spread over me.

Going at a cheetah's pace, I was running so fast in this new metropolitan city that I never stopped to consider why I kept competing and performing to the point of nausea. Who was I trying to impress, my parents once again? Long forgotten faces that told me I wasn't good enough? Like the woman at the Co-op meeting said, forgiveness was on the table, and I had to partake in it or I would lose myself in this fairyland city like so many of its inhabitants. Until I allowed myself a moment to hit the pause button and reflect, I didn't realize how much anger had been festering and boiling deep inside me. As I squeezed the woman's hands—my only link to the real world—an unpredictable cry spewed forth. It was more out of embarrassment that I kept apologizing to the woman for crying. She assured me it was all right, and I believed her.

At that point, I didn't know how to arrive at the distant land called Forgiveness. I didn't know if I should call and tell my brother, Finger, Karen, Raven, Pop, and even God that I forgave them. Saying a couple of rosaries at the nearby church seemed like a good idea, but I quickly changed my mind. Those avenues seemed too trite, too sophomoric. There had to be some other way.

Where do I start?

36 Yank

To appear in a play, any member of Co-op could audition for the role they desired—just because we were members didn't mean we were guaranteed roles. This healthy competition upped the ante, and since most of the actors in Co-op were seasoned performers, I had to be on my game with no room for mistakes if I wanted a part. Since living in L.A. for three years, competition had grown to be my greatest motivator.

The first play that grabbed my interest was the opener for the 2001-2002 season, a show that would affect me in a most profound way. Written in the forties and set in the throes of World War II, *The Hasty Heart* centers around a band of injured Allied soldiers—an Australian, a Brit, a New Zealander, a Scot, and an American Southerner—who battle their fears and find their lost humanities in the confines of a Burmese infirmary. The whole premise of loyalty and loving thy neighbor attracted me to the piece. Since the play called for actors my age and a plethora of accents, I sprung at the chance. The play was a stutterer's paradise.

Whenever I read a play, I acted out the dialogue by myself. This benefited me in many ways. I would get a sense of the writer's rhythm, and at the same time I would understand the characters in a more subjective light. My excitement with *The Hasty Heart* soon dissipated when I read the play for the first time and came upon some disturbing details. Besides having the most well written lines and a stirring character arc, the Southerner in the play—known as Yank—was written as a stutterer. Re-reading *The Hasty Heart* twice after, I realized Yank's dialogue had a similar pattern as my damaged voice. Uttering dialogue that reflected my impediment forced me to rehash harsh memories. As I tried to block out those memories linked to my stuttering, the voice reappeared. *"Forgive."* I started to loathe that damn voice.

Diligently, I rehearsed every nuance and every dialect for the international roles, while keeping a football field distance away from Yank. The role felt too burdensome and too taxing on my emotions. I chose to hide behind the foreign parts instead. On the day of auditions, I entered the theater fully prepared. After performing the scenes with a variety of foreign accents, I stared out into the mostly vacant seats, waiting for the director's input. Instead, the director asked me the unthinkable, "Could you come back tomorrow night and read for the role of Yank?"

I don't remember agreeing with the director, or walking out of the theater and making my way to the car while a baffling haze filled my head. All I recall is sitting in my Camry and staring at the steering wheel. Could I muster enough courage to tackle the role of a stutterer? Even with a Southern accent, I had to learn another stutterer's rhythm while keeping my own impediment on a short leash. I had spent a lifetime immersing myself in roles to forget myself, and now I faced a role that exposed an intimate facet of me. Despite my dread to reveal and indulge in the similarities between Yank and me, something in my core urged me to embrace the challenge. If I stopped now, then everything I had worked so vehemently to attain would be for naught. Besides, no one in the Co-op could possibly know the heart and soul of a stutterer like me. The responsibility lay heavily upon my shoulders. I had to forge ahead.

After staying up all night preparing for Yank's selected scenes, I gave one of the best auditions I had ever delivered. To my surprise, when I allowed myself to stutter on stage, I felt freer and had more room to take chances. Because Yank and I had a deep connection, there was a sense of comfort that settled into my performance. As a result, the director cast me in the role. The vulnerability and intimacy I had with Yank navigated me through the audition, and ultimately through rehearsals. Soon, art would reflect life as the character unearthed a forgotten side of me.

In the play, Lachie, a newly-admitted temperamental and disgruntled patient, causes conflict in the infirmary by his contemptuous ways. Predictably, the men don't like their new Scottish bunkmate. Unbeknownst to Lachie, the men are notified that Lachie may die from his kidney injury, and the men, led by Yank, put their grievances aside and make Lachie's last days as comfortable and joyous as possible. Casting aside his jaded temperament and defenses, the Scot ultimately gives in and finds peace through Yank's heroism, friendship, and patience. Representing the quintessential soldier who adheres to self-sacrifice and who resists the urge to hide away like most stutters are inclined to do, Yank dedicates his life to care for those in need, even when he runs the risk of being rejected.

These virtuous ideals in Yank compelled me to question the reasoning behind my own life's pursuits. As long as I could remember, I tried to prove my self-worth to others through my accomplishments, never putting anyone or anything else above my neediness to be the best boy and the perfect man in the eyes of everyone. Was this the driving force behind my unrelenting quest in L.A.? To say I told you so? Was it a form of vengeance, a form of needy acceptance?

The war I waged against words I did alone, hardly ever allowing anyone truly in. Even with the Knott's boys, I never let them enter my guarded walls, into the attic of my being that housed a boy with an injured voice. According to my distorted reality, the countless faces I encountered every day would sooner or later abandon me, or take advantage of me if they discovered my broken side. Instead, I put on a grand spectacle, starring Rooster as the lead, or any other superficial personality I could create or portray. Still, in my late twenties, I continued to embody the leading man syndrome on a more complicated level.

Backstage one night as I repeated Yank's emotional monologue to myself before going on stage, a memory filtered back—a memory that only a guy like Yank could force me to tap into. There was a kid at my high school named Will. His demeanor and the way he spoke hinted that he was undoubtedly different than the testosterone-laden boys who shuffled through the halls of Rummel High School. Some would call Will "Faggot," "Prissy," and other euphemisms that reflected homophobia. To say I never participated in such name-callings behind Will's back would have been a lie. But on some random day during my senior year, I would redeem myself.

After one of my morning classes, I came around the corner of a hallway. Pressed against the lockers, Will was surrounded by three seniors. As I drew nearer, I could see a pair of hands pressing on Will, as one of them taunted him, "I bet you peek at all of us showering after PE, huh?"

My instincts kicked in and I balked, "H-Hey, l-leave him a-a-alone."

The bullies caught sight of me. "Screw off, stutterbird, this don't concern you."

But they were wrong. This did concern me. I didn't know what kind of retribution awaited me from the three bulky masses, but I stood firm and held my ground. Waiting for what felt like forever, I anticipated two outcomes; they would either leave or pounce on me. To my surprise, they did the former, but not without a derogatory parting shot, "Maybe y'all should go take showers together, you theater faggots."

Wiping his face as his offenders walked away, Will turned his thankful eyes towards me. I asked if he was all right. He nodded. I could tell he was lying. To calm his nerves, I proceeded to tell him about my many encounters with bullies, and how I felt as if my fists were constantly raised every day. I don't know why, but my mouth went a mile a minute as I regurgitated all my daily dreads, while Will leaned on the lockers and simply listened to me. The conversation lasted five minutes, yet in those few moments I found peace. At first my intervention was intended to help a soul in need. But inadvertently, I was really helping myself.

Whether we want to admit it or not, a stutterer tows a hero complex around his neck like a precious chain. Only problem is, we tend to hide that chain under our thick layers, and asking for help seems unfathomable in our "I-can-do-it-on-my-own" state of mind. But sometimes heroes need saving, too.

Beyond my portrayal of Yank, the future roles that awaited me didn't serve to satisfy my ego—the one thing that craved acceptance and perfection. Not anymore. Instead, my acting achievements were for the millions out there who wanted to be heard, wanted to make that appearance on stage, just like the stuttering boy from Metairie who still felt trapped and insignificant in his impediment. And maybe as I turned my suffering into a blessing, perhaps I would find forgiveness, allow myself to be imperfect, and—like Ross the Baker--in that imperfection, perhaps I could find my perfection.

For as long as I could remember, I always wanted to be part of a story bigger than me.

37 Going the Distance

"To sustain longevity, you have to evolve."
—Aries Spears

Once *The Hasty Heart* opened, it was an instant hit for the Co-op, and inaugurated me into a theater company that became my conservatory, as well as my sanctuary for the next six years. From the sociopath Roat in *Wait Until Dark* to the maniacal Pedro in *Man of La Mancha*, I relished in each performance, and thanked God every day for opportunity to say words, even if most of the roles asked for an accent. When I took an extended leave of absence from Co-op in the fall of 2006, I had ten plays under my belt. To this day, I still reflect upon my time at Co-op with heartwarming gratitude.

A week after we closed *Hasty Heart* in late 2001, I got the call. "Is this Scott Damian?" asked the youthful voice on the other end.

"This is he," I replied, presuming the call was some random sales scheme. I was happily proven wrong when the voice introduced herself as Kim, owner of a prosperous boutique talent agency in L.A.

"I saw your performance in *The Hasty Heart* last week and I'd like to call you in for an interview. Are you signed with anyone?"

I told her no, so Kim suggested we meet the following week. After hanging up with Karen, I laughed at the irony of it all. My portrayal of a stutterer—the very role I tried so desperately to distance myself from—attracted an L.A. agent. Mazel Tov, Yank.

That next week, I showed up promptly at Kim's office—a cozy bungalow just north of Universal Studios. A respected agent who was an ordained preacher on the side, Kim looked forty, maybe forty-five, yet her youthful demeanor and sincerity were the first things that attracted me during our meeting. I'd heard many horror stories of agents conning desperate actors, yet Kim seemed like the antithesis of a sleazy type. Besides, she was a preacher for a local Presbyterian church, so what harm could she do?

"I wasn't taking on any new clients, but I'm really interested in you," she said. "Quite frankly, we need to build up your credits, but I think you can do well here. You're very talented."

I smiled and thanked her. Most of the conversation consisted of her talking and me listening. As much as she made me feel at ease, I was hesitant to share my speech impediment with her. To do so would probably sabotage my one shot at signing with an agent. As our meeting wrapped up and she offered me a contract, I decided not to tell her about my apprehensions regarding my voice. It was my secret battle. I'd take care of it like I always did in the past.

Auditioning for TV and film is a daunting beast, especially for a stutterer. Because everything happens at a high-velocity rate, a stutterer's anxiety can reach paramount proportions if he or she isn't prepared mentally. Being off book, crafty, creative, and skilled in cold reading—meaning looking at a scene for a few minutes and performing it like it's second nature—are essential tools to an actor's success.

From 2002 to 2004—before emails and texts were of mandatory use between agent and client—my audition process went something like this: I received a page from Kim's office in the late afternoon or early evening. Calling back, Kim's assistant would tell me, "They want to see you at 10:30 A.M. on Warner Brothers' lot." At that point I had to find some competent individual to cover my shift at Knott's for the next day, go pick up a copy of the scenes from my agent's office clear across town before they closed, study and prepare the material late into the night, get up two hours before my audition, staple my picture and resume together, battle fickle morning L.A. traffic, make my way through the maze of a studio lot, and then perform a lasting impression on a tired, caffeinated casting director, while thirty competent actors—who were vying for the same role— waited impatiently outside the casting office. It was a fast moving, almost farcical train, and if I wasn't on my game, I'd probably land flat on my ass.

Fortunately, because of my black hair, olive complexion, and Mediterranean features, the roles that I was initially called in for ranged from Sicilian mobster to Armenian hit man. I had a chance to dig deep into my bag of accents and rummage through it, until I found the one that best suited the character. The fear of exposing my stuttering to high profile producers and casting directors were kept to a minimum. Even though filming shorts with the Knott's boys proved my ability to say lines in front of a camera while using my natural voice, I still carried a pensive feeling when confronting high-ranking Hollywood types.

In 2003, I landed my first TV spot as a French art collector on ABC's soap opera, *Port Charles*. As a theater actor who had never been on a television stage before, to do a one-liner on daytime television was like winning an Emmy. Yes, to some it may have been perceived as petty, saying six words in a French accent—"Hew mooch iz diz pes werrth?" (Translation: How much is this piece worth?)—but the thought of a stutterer standing on a soundstage with bright lights peering down, and three cameras directed at him, was an inconceivable notion at one time. So I allowed myself to relish in the experience.

An hour after Kim informed me of my soap opera gig, I called Momma and Pop. Momma was ecstatic. Pop, on the other hand, gave his best rendition of congratulations and finished up with, "Just don't sign anything unless you really, really read it. They'll screw you over."

The filming of a soap opera moves faster than a tap dancer's feet. You rehearse the scene as the director blocks you on where to go. After blocking, you go to makeup, then to wardrobe, wait for an hour in your dressing room before they call you to the set. Depending on the amount of dialogue, a typical soap opera scene films for ten to thirty minutes. Because of deadlines, an actor must be fully prepared for anything. It could cost thousands of wasted dollars because of one hiccup. If an actor is the cause of that glitch, he or she is instantly branded as a problem. And when you're trying to build a viable reputation as a newcomer, you want your record as clean as your grandmother's best crystal.

Before my feet hit the studio parking lot that morning, I made sure those six words were second nature to me, including a French accent that resembled Peter Sellers in *The Pink Panther*. Once they called my name over the speakers asking me to report to the soundstage, I made my way from my dressing room to the set while repeating the lines aloud.

A constant worry followed me onto the set, similar to when I walked onto the Genesian stage for the first time, or when I opened my mouth to say that first word of dialogue as Herodias. Would I stammer? Would I make a fool of myself? Would I halt production because of my impediment?

Even though the shoot went well, and the popular soap star I acted opposite said, "Nice job, kid," I still held some skepticism about my future once I left the studio. Perhaps this was just a one-time deal. Maybe I couldn't book a "next" role, especially in my own voice. Sensing an immense challenge approaching, I knew the day would come—like in Ian's class—when I'd be obligated to use my own voice in an audition, or worse, on a television and film set in front of producers, writers, and other powerful people who held my fate in their hands.

"They want to see you again this afternoon," Kim said to me over the phone. "But they want you to lose that whatever-accent you're doing. Can you do that?" I almost dropped the phone when I heard the cataclysmic request.

The "they" Kim referred to was the casting director, writers, executive producer and director of the popular NBC show, *Las Vegas*. In its second season, the show centered around Ed, the casino manager, starring James Caan, and Danny, his young, hip, head of security, played by Josh Dummel, as they navigate through the slimy world of Las Vegas while successfully operating a casino called the Monticello. When I initially went into read for the prime time show, I had a heavy Brooklyn accent already in place for an unctuous Internet pimp who rented out his girls online.

Dressing the part, and preparing my best thick New York accent, I made sure my lines had intention. For the initial audition, my intent was to bring a realistic element to my character without being overly sleazy. In front of a camcorder, I said my three pages of lines for the casting director in her tiny office. She thanked me, and I exited the office, thinking all went swimmingly. But after my agent's call for the callback, all bets were off the table. I had a new dragon to conquer.

The following day, my breathing came at short bursts as I paced in the waiting room of the casting office. Two other nervous actors sat near me. Between the three of us, one would win the prize as Stanley, and the remaining two would have to deal with another rejection.

Glancing down at the lines, the bad no-no's leaped off the page and chiseled away at my confidence. How the hell could I say these lines without my crutch, without some form of accent? In my head, I replaced one word with another, and then another. Before I knew it, I was rewriting my lines. Paraphrasing was my only hope; I was out of options.

Rushing out of the room, I made my way to a more secluded part of the hallway. I had to get my head straight. There was no way I could make up lines when the writer would be sitting in the same room. Crouching down in a corner, I closed my eyes. Our Father's and Hail Mary's filtered out of my mouth. As I prayed to God for some morsel of relief, I saw him — Will's face looking at me from so many years ago. Then it hit me all at once. The white knight resurfaced, but he wasn't there to take me away from the situation. On the contrary, he showed up to remind me of why I fought so arduously.

In that hallway, I smacked the wall. I was tired of the lies, tired of being perfect, even for people I hardly knew. I had a right to be there, not because some casting director deemed it so, but because I had paid my dues, and because God put me in that situation for a reason.

Returning to the waiting area, I scanned the room, studying the actors' faces once again. But this time my perception of them changed; they were no longer a threat to my immediate future. My will was firm, and my stance resolute. I was going to book this job, not for me, but for the boy inside of me who had been knocked around for too long by his perpetual tormentor. This was for that kid, for Will, for Pauley, for Ross the Baker, and for all of those like us.

I heard my name called. Tucking the pages into my back pocket, I entered the office, greeted the creative staff, and waited for the casting director to give me the cue line. The four faces staring back at me didn't resemble the intimidating gods I imagined them to be. Instead, I saw my Knott's buddies; Eddie, Rich, Cola, and Matt behind the table, with Aaron aiming the camcorder at me. In that brief moment, I was filming with the boys.

When the cue line came from the casting director, I went for it. Supported by my diaphragm, the words eased out, no accent, all confidence, and all from memory. After that first line, the rest of the words connected. Like a track runner, I hurdled over the bad no-no's.

Finishing my last line, I broke out of the moment. There was a long silence. The director whispered to the writer. Looking away from the writer, the director asked me, "Could you do the scene again, but this time, make it more...urgent."

"Certainly," I replied. Anyway they wanted it, I'd give it to them in my own God-given voice. No more would I run away.

38 I'm Ready For My Close Up, Mr. Corleone

"My acting technique is to look up at God just before the camera rolls, and say, 'Give me a break.'"
—James Caan

He had that swagger where the chest protruded out, arms swayed back and forth behind him, part John Wayne, and part James Cagney—all man. The intensity in his face reminded me of a street brawler. When he strolled onto the set that Friday morning at the Culver City studios, James Caan owned the room. Every grip and technician stopped what they were doing and greeted him. "Hey, James!" and "Morning Mr. Caan" echoed throughout the set that looked like a rundown, low-end office where only a pimp could reside. Patiently, I waited to introduce myself as James Caan came closer. I couldn't come across as too star struck or too enthusiastic. He was the mayor, and I was just a visitor to his fair town.

After our formal introductions, we got down to business. Taking our places, the director staged the scene. Once Caan said a certain line, I was to rise from behind the desk and deliver the rest of my lines, spewing off information on where to find a certain prostitute. It would be simple, an easy back and forth. *Should be in and out in an hour*, I thought.

During our rehearsal, I found myself trying to lock eyes with Caan, striving to make a connection from one actor to the other. An older version of Caan stared back at me, but his blue rimmed eyes still looked the same; those intense, antagonizing bulbs that reminded me of his former self, his Sonny Corleone.

The persona of Sonny followed James in every part he portrayed, representing the ultimate volatile macho man. For me, James and Sonny were synonymous.

The days leading up to filming our scene, I worked out the lines in my head, and those of Caan and Josh Dummel's as well. I knew the scene backwards and forwards, nothing was getting past me. Since Kim's call telling me that I booked the part, I had one terrifying thought—James Caan would lose his temper because of my imperfect voice, and my possible mishaps on set. So, to balance out this fear, I was motivated to be the consummate professional. As I'd experienced many times before, familiarity was a stutterer's friend, and going over my lines and rehearsing every movement—where to place my hand on a certain line, or how to gesture on another—helped solidify a confidence.

To my relief, our rehearsal went smoothly, just a casual layout of what the scene would ultimately be. After James grunted a "See ya soon" to me, I left the rehearsal and headed out. Returning to my trailer—which was the size of a washing machine—I encountered one of the assistant directors (AD) waiting for me at the trailer door.

"Hey, Scott, we got rewrites for you. Hot off the press." He handed me four pink pages of dialogue. "If you have any questions, let me know. I know on the first page and on the last page they rewrote a lot of your lines. You can handle it, right?"

Forcing a smile, I lied. "Sure."

"Cool, I'll come getcha in a half hour. They should be ready for you on set by then."

Hopping in his cart, the AD puttered away, leaving me to brew in my new predicament. Familiarity vacated the premise, and I was left with a gripping insecurity. Perusing through the pages, I heard the frequent lie in my head once again; *You're going to fail. No one is going to like you. Just be quiet.*

Rewrites at the last minute are part of show business. The writer may have an epiphany the night before, and he'll rearrange plot points or clean up dialogue that sounds too artificial. Sometimes the director or producer catches a flaw in the scene and requests a rewrite. Or celebrities may want more lines or fewer lines, depending on his or her mood, which may include their occasional hangover from the night before. There are a plethora of reasons for last minute rewrites, but for an actor who is outside of the celebrity realm, none of these reasons matter. We must say the given lines regardless. It is part of the job description to learn lines, learn them fast, and have the right objective behind them, no questions asked.

Memorizing lines was a forced habit I learned long ago to ease the pressure from my erratic voice. If I didn't see the words on the page, I wouldn't notice the bad no-no's as much, giving me a greater chance to speak them clearly. But with the arrival of rewrites on my trailer doorstep, I had a laborious half hour ahead of me. As I read through the lines, the habitual urge for perfection beat in my chest. My hands shook. I couldn't stop fidgeting. There were no accents to depend on. To severely stutter in front of Sonny Corleone was an unfathomable notion, yet now it all seemed like a probable outcome.

An hour later, I took my mark behind the desk. The new lines stampeded through my memory. The lines didn't feel organic; they felt superficial. I hadn't mastered them yet. I mouthed them to myself, until the director said, "Action." Lights beamed down as James Caan approached me. Just two feet behind Caan, I could see Josh Dummel taking his mark. The camera was over my shoulder, getting Caan's reaction shots first. James said his first line, which was my cue. Taking a deep breath, I tried to say one of the newly written lines in my cadence, but my mouth didn't follow suit. A sound similar to a helicopter propeller puttered out of my mouth. I focused too much on the outcome instead of just being in the moment. It didn't help to have an agitated James Caan in front of me—who probably hemmed and hawed about the rewrites. I wanted to please and to be liked—the worse two predicaments for any stutterer. To dodge this embarrassing moment, I waved my hands in the air and played it off like I forgot my line.

"Sorry," I said, acting better in real life than in the scene.

"Cut!" said the director.

"You okay?" asked Caan as the crew reset for another take.

"Yes, sir, Mr. Caan."

"No need to call me sir. Jimmy is fine. Listen, I'm going to try something here, so you just play along, okay?"

"Sure," I replied, relieved that quite possibly James Caan and I had an unsaid relationship, and a shared mission to make this a perfect scene. A great warmth of comfort slid over me. Suddenly, the tension left my body, and my playful side resurfaced, just like all those times I filmed guerrilla style with the boys. I had Mayor Caan on my side. I wasn't alone after all.

The director ordered us to go again. Caan said my cue line, but before I could dwell too much on my apprehensions, Caan grabbed the prop computer from off the desk, picked it up and chucked it onto the floor. I jumped back, unaware of his impromptu action. I loved the spontaneity that was all Caan. Instantly, I flowed with whatever the veteran actor was giving me. I reacted to Caan's aggressiveness; it gave me more to play with and distracted me from my fears. Finally, I had something to play off of. I wasn't Scott anymore; I was acting as Stanley, the Internet pimp. From then on, the scene popped, and our snappy rhythm continued for two more successful takes as the new lines poured out of my mouth.

As the crew prepared for the reverse shot—which would be my reaction shot—the actors and I took a ten-minute break. The director approached me as I munched on some carrots at the craft service table. I was feeling more confident about the scene, so I expected praise for our performances. Whispering in my ear like a conspirator, the director asked, "Hey listen, can you not react and pause when James throws the computer? In fact, don't even wait for him to throw the computer. Just keep going with the dialogue. Yes?"

Nodding in approval, I asked the director, "D-Did you tell James?"

"No, just do it. The camera is on you anyway so we won't get Jimmy's reaction." Before I could express my concern, the director ducked behind the corner and was gone. But even if I wanted to express my reservations, I wouldn't. I was the new kid on the block. I didn't want to create waves, not with the director, or with James Caan. I felt pulled in two different directions. Do I abide with the director's request, or do I stand up for our scene? *Be a good boy*, I reminded myself.

Returning to set, the director bellowed out, "Action!" Our scene began like before. Before Caan had a chance to clutch the computer and chug it, I cut him off with my line. "I-I-I d-dont..." The stuttering came up again because the moment felt synthetic— something was off, something unexplainable. Suddenly, James's face turned beat red right in front of me. His eyes morphed into the same razor-sharp glare he had when portraying Sonny Corleone. "Cut!" Caan screamed.

Flabbergasted, I stood still, unable to move. Caan leaned into me. "Did you switch shit up on me, or did the director make you do it?"

I couldn't tell a lie even if I tried. Court was in session and James Caan wasn't the mayor anymore, he was the goddamn jury. I said my peace, "No, James, he asked me to ch-change it up and to just go right through..."

Caan didn't need to hear anymore. Like a lion about to pounce, the veteran actor turned and yelled for the director. Sheepishly, the director came from around the corner with a concerned look on his face. The gazelle knew something was up. "What's wrong, Jimmy?"

"Don't Jimmy me, it's Mr. Caan to you!" James said in a ferocious voice that made everyone stop and observe the event unfolding. Gaffers, sound guys, even Josh stood at attention as James continued, "Did you make this kid change our established scene?" Before the director could respond, James laid into him further, "What kind of director switches up a scene after they set the timing and action in the first shots? It's called continuity! What are you trying to do here?"

The director muttered, "I'm sorry."

"Sorry?" asked Jimmy in a rhetorical fashion. "Well, this kid and I had a good thing going on, so do you mind if we continue with it?" Caan wasn't asking, he was ordering.

"Certainly...yes, you just do whatever you want," said the director. Trying to gain some type of authority to his embarrassing situation, the director ducked out of sight while saying over his shoulder, "Okay, let's go back to one, and do it like before, guys. It looks great."

Snickering, James turned to face me. His triumphant face said it all.

"So, how should I do this?" I asked in a whisper.

"We do it our way, kid," Caan replied. "Don't let them tell you how to do it. Trust yourself, you know more than you think."

As I took in Caan's words, a shot of adrenaline pumped through me. I was ready to tackle the scene fearlessly because Sonny Corleone was on my side. Like a tango, we had perfected a dance between us. The stuttering and insecurities that came with the rewrites took a back seat. I had a right to be under the lights, in front of the camera, and in the midst of a legend like James Caan. "You're doing good, just play it like before," Caan said before we started the scene. He winked at me. I winked back. The director called for action.

39 Hurricane Season

"When words are both true and kind, they can change the world."
—Buddha

It took a while to process the events that occurred on August 29, 2005. Seeing my hometown engulfed in eighteen feet of water spun me into a state of helplessness. I couldn't fly out to New Orleans at a moment's notice. Airports were closed, roads were blocked, and nothing was allowed in or out of the city. Besides, my parents weren't home. Like most of the inhabitants in the Gulf region, my family joined the great exodus days prior to the hurricane's arrival.

All I could do was watch the images plastered across the TV screen that showed the aftermath of Hurricane Katrina—floating bodies, Rummel's football field turned triage center, destroyed bridges and freeways that looked like scattered Legos. Like stumbling into *The Matrix* after swallowing the red pill, things that were familiar became unfamiliar to me.

I waited impatiently for my family to call. When they did, the conversation was like something out of a melodrama; the strain and desperation in their voices seeped out of the receiver. Cooped up in an Alabama hotel, Momma shared her thoughts, "Everything is probably gone, baby." She tried to hold back the tears, tried to appear resilient, like all parents must do in front of their children.

Then Pop got on the phone. "I don't know, son. I don't know…" he kept repeating. Pop's shaky voice threw me for a loop. It didn't carry the stoutness and certainty he had garnered from years of hardship. Twice prior I had heard Pop's quivering voice, on the brink of tears. Once when he laid his mother to rest in New Orleans, and the other, when we visited his father's grave in Guatemala.

But when I heard Pop's trembling timbre over the phone, I knew nothing would be the same, not within my familial dynamics, and not in the city that I once called home. Mother Nature's hand changed my father, my mother, and countless others forever, including me. Listening to Pop, I was reminded of the verse from Scripture: "The first shall be last, and the last shall be first."

Whether we want to admit it or not, stutterers are hypersensitive beings. Acute awareness of our emotions and others' emotions are a by-product of the impediment. This emotional awareness is fine-tuned from studying the responses of people when we stammer, from the introspection we force ourselves into due to our silence, and from the development of an in-depth empathy for others who suffer just like us. As we grow older and our sensibilities are sharpened, we become pseudo-analysts, or in my case, an actor and writer. In my family, I would soon become the emotional thinker, the perspective keeper who pointed out the unmentionables and all the unsaid issues that plagued not only me, but my family as well.

With the devastation of Katrina, the gritty and honest aspects of my family were unearthed and brought to the surface as they relentlessly spun through my head: My parents' dispassionate marriage—how they never showed affection to one another and how, recently, their emotional distance continued by both Momma and Pop residing in different bedrooms—and the addictions that ran rampant through our family, which included Momma Nettie's dependence on alcohol, Momma's constant anxiety that she was never enough and that the world punishes those who are abandoned and imperfect, Pop's addiction to work and constant perfection as he tried to embody the American Dream, and my brother's need to be recognized, revered, and praised for the artificial persona that he had created.

Even when I was too young to comprehend the significance of my family's brokenness, I felt it internally, yet could never communicate it. For me, it was palpable as the unsaid pressed heavily upon my heart. And even if I wanted to express how I felt about my family as I grew older, I couldn't. We never discussed such matters in our house. Like any house that preached the baby-boomer mantra "things are the way they are, so let's not discuss, and just live with it," my house never over-analyzed the issues in which each of us silently suffered. We kept a tight lip about our problems, as everyone played his or her parts, coping the best way we could.

Maybe my stuttering was linked to my family's practiced silence when it came to dysfunctional matters. Perhaps as I got older, I wanted to yell, scream, and point out the elephant in the room, yet my shame and guilt to even consider my family as frail and fallible strangled me by sub-consciously perpetuating a speech impediment.

To this day, I still don't know if there is a direct correlation between my familial issues and my stuttering, but during those days in September of 2005, I knew something wasn't right in my family. It hadn't been for a long time. I couldn't stay silent any longer. I had to dig deeper and, for the first time, express it. My life depended on it.

For weeks, my family's dysfunctions filtered through my head as I rustled some sort of logic behind them. Begrudgingly, I accepted them—faults and all—because they reminded me of who I was, who I am, and who I wanted to be. Like the inhabitants in the Gulf region, I leaped into my own toxic waters of the past and tirelessly swam through them, searching for my way back home.

I stared at the bright monitor of my laptop. The digital clock on the screen said: 1:11A.M., 9/10/05. I had no idea why I rose from my bed, stumbled my way to the desk, and flipped on the laptop. The words were in my head, and they had to be released. I typed the first word, a word that evolved into a line of dialogue. Dialogue became scenes. Scenes eventually became acts. The words derived from a different plain; instinctually, they regurgitated out of me because— like my relationship with storytelling many times before—I needed words to save me.

A few months later, I gave birth to a play titled, *Coffee Stains*. The play takes place days and hours before the arrival of Hurricane

Katrina. Set in the kitchen of a family-owned New Orleans restaurant, a volatile family comes to terms with their fragile identities and their deep-rooted lies, as they finally let go of their facades, their secrets, and their prestigious reputations. The emotional storm brewing in the family is only paralleled by the violent hurricane that is about to make landfall. For me, the play was a cathartic release that seeped out from the pores of my past. In the course of writing it, I found peace and an unrivaled security in my voice, not only in my written words, but in my spoken words as well.

Writing the play was one journey, perfecting it became another. Working and reworking the play in casual readings, my play morphed into a story that many related to in various ways. After the readings, and during informal talkbacks, some viewers and members of the cast shared their stories and the dysfunctions that plagued their own families. For a stutterer, to create words and characters that resonated with others was something that exceeded anything I had ever accomplished. My words became their words. Finally, I had found a new endeavor to release the emotions steeping inside of me. But like many aspirations, I found resistance along the way from those closest to me.

. Two Christmases after Katrina, my brother and I were standing in the middle of my parent's kitchen. Twenty-eight months had passed since the hurricane, and my parent's house had remained unscathed. It was the first time we'd gathered as a family since the storm. But on one particular night, I found my brother confrontational—his hand glued to his hips and a scowl arched on his face.

Throwing the pages of my play onto the countertop, my brother grunted, "I just read your play."

The house had been quiet until his voice shook the kitchen. His wife and three kids were fast asleep, as well as my parents who called it a night two hours prior.

"Oh yeah, what'd you think?" I asked, sipping on my hot coco. I knew his answer would be lathered in criticism. My brother drew closer. "You can never publish your play. You know that, right?"

I slammed my mug down. "Who says? You? It's my p-play. It's my words, and I can do whatever the hell I want with it."

"That play is about our family, isn't it?"

"Well, that's your interpretation," I replied, feeling my temper rising. In that moment, my eyes caught a glimmer of my parents' bookshelf in the living room. On it were two of my brother's best-selling books. From actor, to journalist, to author, my brother had covered a gambit of careers. As I stood in the kitchen, I realized my brother wasn't concerned about the family name. He probably saw me as a threat. No more was I a silent kid, a gypsy, or a stuttering buffoon. I had something profound to say, and I may have been damn good at saying it. Even as adults, I could see that sibling rivalry still thrived between two grown men.

But I didn't need his approval. All my life, I'd stayed silent, while craving favor from people I didn't know and from others who didn't believe in me. Wasted years were spent on useless validation; not realizing the only validation I needed came from me.

I suddenly felt calm. "You and no one else will ever keep me quiet."

In a huff, my brother turned and walked away. Like the Chihuahua that chased me in the backyard when I was six, my brother's bark was bigger than his bite. But this time, I confronted the bark. It would be the last disconcerting thing my brother said about my play, or any of my other projects. I wouldn't talk to him for another two years.

40 For Us

"When his parents saw him, they were overwhelmed. His mother said to him, 'Child, why have you treated us like this? Look, your father and I have been looking for you anxiously.' But he replied, 'Why were you looking for me?'"
—Luke: 48-49

Marking the four-year anniversary of Hurricane Katrina in September of 2009, my play found its way to the Zephyr Theater off Melrose Ave. It was the first professional reading for the play where investors, playwrights, producers, and celebrities filled the theater for two nights. That first night was just as important to me as if we premiered it at the Nederlander in New York.

During the development of a play, professional readings are essential to make a script as polished as possible. Some readings are done where the actors sit in a semi-circle and just read the text aloud. Others—like the one we elected for our play—have the actors move on stage with emotional intentions while holding their scripts. The reason behind these readings is for the writer and producer to hear the words, see the play up on its feet, and gauge the audience's responses. How my play arrived at a place where proficient actors invested their time and energy into my words wasn't just by my doing alone, but by the grace of God, and the efforts of a producer named Heather Provost.

Meeting in the most auspicious of circumstances in 2004— before Heather put her photographic memory and her keen business sense to better use as a producer—Heather and I performed together at Universal Studios Hollywood in a live high-action rock n' roll show that merged singing with stunts to the mythology of Spiderman called *Spiderman Rocks*. During rehearsals and throughout the two-year run of *Spiderman Rocks*, Heather and I forged a unique bond. Call it a Sicilian bond or an instant attraction where both parties perceive one another's loyalties and future successes — I as a writer and she as a sought after Broadway producer.

The road to get *Coffee Stains* to a showcase level was an arduous task, to say the least. Two days before our sold-out reading, we battled resistance that came in the form of a pretentious director and the neurotic tendencies of a celebrity actor and actress. Replacing the director a week before opening, as well as our two leading actors twenty-four hours before the reading kept us on our toes. Yet we prevailed, and everyone, from cast to crew, rose to the occasion. Our mutual respect and trust for one another — which is a rare commodity in our business — as well as our faith and commitment to my words guided Heather and me in finding a solution. And to have someone like Heather protect and defend my voice in Hollywood was something I couldn't have imagined from anyone.

As the Sunday night audience filtered into the Zephyr Theater, Heather and I took our seats in the last row. As the lights dimmed in the house, my parents sat up straighter in their seats. They had accumulated more gray since the last time I'd seen them, and they were no doubt exhausted from their flight from New Orleans to L.A. But they were here for my big night.

The lights came up on stage. I held my breath. It would be the first time my parents witnessed my play live on stage; a play that my folks inspired more than they realized. As the play proceeded, an all-too-familiar insecurity crept up inside of me. Suddenly, I was a boy again, wondering if my parents would approve of my work, and if they would look at me as a success. I grew annoyed with myself for having such a resurgence of childhood doubts.

After the play, Momma startled me as she snuck up behind me in the lobby. She wrapped her warm arms around my waist and kissed me. I turned and embraced her. The sweat and tears from her cheek moistened my face. I'd missed those kisses. Over the loud banter from the post-show soirée, Momma was ecstatic. "That was beautiful, baby. I loved it."

After a few more accolades, Momma told me Pop went to the bathroom, so I took the opportunity to ask her how he liked the play. She shrugged and said she didn't know.

Pointing behind her, Momma asked if she could meet a celebrity who starred in her favorite sitcom. Ten hours in L.A. and Momma was already star-struck. I held Momma's hand and led her to the gracious celebrity, who promptly took a liking to my mother. To my surprise, they both clicked, and I gawked from afar, elated to see the excited little girl come out of Momma. So far, L.A. was jelling well with her. That was when the familiar voice from behind me said, "Son."

I swiveled around, and there stood Pop, his eyes beat red, and his cheeks rosy behind his tan complexion. *Had he been crying?* I wondered as we hugged. Instantly, I was propelled back to that fifteen-year-old who'd just come off stage from performing *Little Shop of Horrors*—a different body, a different man, yet the same yearning for acceptance. Does it ever go away?

"Really good job, son...I ah..." Suddenly, Pop searched for words as his eyes danced from side to side. "That's our family up there, huh?" asked Pop, pointing his thumb back to the theater.

"Well, it wasn't exactly like our family, Pop, but the heart and soul of our family is there. You, me, Momma..."

Interrupting me, Pop said, "I thought so." The tremble in his voice couldn't be ignored. He had an emotional build-up stirring behind his brown eyes. Averting his attention to the ground, Pop muttered something that I never would've predicted. "Your words...they were...beautiful." A drip or two fell from his eyes. He tried to stealthily wipe them away, but he couldn't hide it from me. It would be the fourth time I heard that vulnerability in my father's voice, and I loved him all the more for that.

Three days after the reading of *Coffee Stains*, I found myself in the pit below another stage, and a much larger theater. Waiting for my cue, I caught my reflection in the clear Plexiglas in front of me. My whole face was covered in blue latex and blue airbrush, resembling a popular Disney icon. In a moment, a hydraulic trap would elevate me onto the stage where I would make a grand entrance as the dramatic music blared and liquid nitrogen puffed from all around me. How I'd gotten to this blessed point in my life was a story in itself.

Four months prior to Katrina, in April of 2005, as I perused through *Backstage West*—a trade paper for actors—a particular breakdown instantly caught my attention: "Announcing Auditions For *Aladdin: A Musical Spectacular* At The Disneyland Resort."

Based on the popular animated film of the same name and geared as a Broadway-bound production, this lavish musical found a permanent home at the Hyperion Theater, a two thousand seat, state-of-the art theater located at Disney California Adventure in Southern California. Glancing through the list of characters, I was certain I had a chance to book one role in particular; the part of the wisecracking parrot, Iago.

Days later, my hand slipped into the intricate puppet that resembled the parrot from the movie. Playing with it for a while, I grew more confident in how to manipulate the puppet. Its beak fit perfectly around my fingers, and the neck had wiggle room for my wrist to animate. The wings flapped with ease. Nothing but confidence exuded from me as I breathed life into the puppet in front of the Disney executives. I had known puppeteering for quite some time, especially from my college summers at Disney, and during my childhood when my brother and I manipulated inanimate objects—from paper bags to socks—into living, breathing characters.

Instead of the conventional way where the puppeteer hides in a pit and extends the puppet out onstage, *Aladdin* brought a revolutionary concept to puppeteering. In their show, both performer and puppet were exposed onstage, moving as one entity. Understanding the concept that it was more about the puppet than about me, I found nuances and details in the audition that I had long forgotten.

After two callbacks, I booked the job and signed a contract with Disney. A one-year contract turned into five more contracts; the part of the parrot was just a gateway to a treasure trove of roles. In the span of three years, I auditioned and booked the role of Genie, Jafar, Sultan, and the Head Guard—each character contrasting in voice, execution, and appearance. Soon, I became principal swing, which in theater terms meant that I'd fill in for the principal performers to help them rest their bodies and voices. Having the chance to play a plethora of roles and switch personalities at a moment's notice was something a stutterer like me never took for granted. Portraying a maniacal bad guy sporting a Standard English tone, or a parrot with a quasi-Gilbert Godfrey voice, or an irreverent blue Genie who sounded like a taxi driver, I enjoyed flipping gears in my physical instruments as well as in my appearance when bringing each character to life.

Some frowned on the job, saying *Aladdin: A Musical Spectacular* was just "a theme park show." Others called it a "wanna-be" Broadway show stuck in Orange County. I saw it in a different light. Having the chance and the ability to say clear, concise words in front of two thousand people every day, and getting paid handsomely for it, wasn't something menial; it was a goddamn miracle for a stutterer. And I couldn't wait to share this unique opportunity with the ones who would appreciate it the most.

In the pit of the Hyperion theater stage, as I felt the blue latex pressing on my forehead, I waited for my entrance. Making the sign of the cross, I offered my performance up to Momma Nettie, like I always did before going on stage. I jabbed at the air like Rocky Balboa as my heart pitter-pattered. I stuck out my tongue, stretching it out; enunciation and commitment to details were my primary goals for the marathon that awaited me. I methodically recited my vowels out loud. I had done this ritual countless times before, but this particular time I had to make certain my intentions were firm because I knew two familiar faces would be watching for the first time.

To my right, a technician nodded his head. I nodded back, letting him know I was ready to go up. I felt the hydraulic system vibrate from underneath me. Like an astronaut, the trap propelled me twelve feet into my own stratosphere and the only galaxy that felt like home.

As the music hit a crescendo, a spotlight hit me center stage. A rowdy applause soon followed with my dramatic introduction. My first line punched out. I was scared, excited, and proud to share this moment with two recognizable eyes staring at me in the front row. This was for them, for the sacrifices they had endured — for Pop, who tirelessly worked under cars and motivated me the only way a once-poor immigrant could; and for Momma, who spent most of her life behind a secretary's desk and her exhausting commitment to find an answer to my impediment. They weren't perfect, but they did the best they could.

Speaking effortlessly, I rejoiced with every bit of dialogue that flowed from my mouth. But this brazen victory not only belonged to my folks in the front row, or to the speaker who uttered them; my stutter-free voice held the essence of those who craved to tear away from their fears and carve a pathway in finding their voices.

This is for you, sweet Ben.

41 And the Beat Goes On...

"The wound is the place where the Light enters you."
—Rumi

Standing in front of the casting director's desk, the stammering comes without warning. I'm not invested in the role, or the two pages of dialogue that are in my right hand. Something else is keeping my mind preoccupied from the audition. I apologize to the casting director and try again. He knows me well enough from previous casting sessions, so his forgiveness is abundant.

"Sure, give it another shot," he says.

Giving the sides a go again, I take in a deep breath and try to utter the first line, but the word still sticks in my throat. Like crashing a party, my impediment barges into the office, enters my being, and has me sounding like a propeller again. Profusely apologizing to the casting director, I ask him if I can take a moment to gather myself. He says of course, and out I go into a secluded area of the waiting room.

Either during auditions or when engaged in normal conversations, my stuttering has been known to make a guest appearance. Still after almost forty years of speaking, the apprehension lingers in the back of my head, wondering if the stuttering will make its way into my mouth. But I have learned not to let it get the best of me. Knowing that advanced preparation is my ally, I still rigorously rehearse my lines before a performance or before an audition so that I keep the stuttering under my thumb. If the stammering does pitter-patter out, I will stop myself, figure out why I'm stuttering, and give it another go. Or when conversing, I'll stumble on a bad no-no occasionally, but it goes undetected by the common listener. Stuttering does not define me any longer; I now define it.

Like fear, the stuttering has become my greatest weapon because it keeps me focused and on my game. Because of my impediment, I have allowed myself to relish in my successes, never taking any advancement for granted. Whether small or monumental, I now share these victories with the ones I love the most, and allow those closest to me into those deep crevices that were once closed off from everyone.

Even though Knott's Berry Farm is far behind us, my band of boys and I still make films together. I am writing consistently, and — as I write this — I have two plays in full development, as well as three screenplays. The joy I now find in creating words and the connection I have with others who suffer — whether it's alcoholism, manic depression, or drug abuses — inspires me to share my story and inadvertently help those who are going through the throes of their own troubles. I celebrate in the scars that we all share. I am one of the sufferers, no better, and no worse.

Every Christmas, I return home to visit my loved ones. When I'm home, Pop and I talk of more constructive things. Since he attended my reading in 2009, we have a better relationship. I guess I made my point by standing my ground and showing my parents that a stuttering boy can make it in the business where words and emotions fuse together.

Every once in a while, my brother visits Los Angeles on business. We'll have lunch, maybe a dinner. It's usually cordial, but there's nothing deep or too earth shattering in our banter. When he brings his kids to California, they usually see the *Aladdin* show. The kids are enthralled with the blue makeup as they poke and feel the latex. After asking a slew of questions about the show, their imaginations run wild. I look on them with fond affection; my two nephews and niece are my brother and I from so long ago. Sometimes, my brother throws in a congratulatory remark on my performance, and I am taken aback by his complement every time. With time and age, sibling rivalry does simmer, I suppose.

When the temperature rises in New Orleans and I'm home for a visit, I'll cut the grass for my folks, reminiscing in my former chores.

The smell of grass and gas emitting from the lawnmower gives me a sentimental satisfaction. I'm that eight-year old again pulling and tugging on the mechanical beast as it slices the monkey grass. Sometimes I see familiar faces pass by the house in the old neighborhood. One face in particular grabs my attention as Mary whisks by the house in her family van. On one random afternoon, Mary decided to stop in front of the house and ask me about L.A., her eyes still beaming that familiar youthfulness. Leaning in her car as we share our "where have you been" moments, I still see that twelve-year old who inspired me to leap into the arena of romanticism. Then reality sets in as I catch a glimpse of the two empty baby car seats in the back of Mary's minivan and a wedding ring that sparkles on her left finger.

Ross still remains The King Baker of Metairie. Picking up an order for Momma for Christmas, I pay Ross and his amazing rolls a visit from time to time. He doesn't remember me in my older version, but that's okay. I remember him; I'll always remember him. He still greets guests with a wave and a stammer, but his stuttering isn't as jarring as before. To me, his voice sounds like poetry.

Every year, I make it a point to sit in front of a mausoleum stone and talk to a special redhead who is still alive in my thoughts. Brass letters appear on the cold slab, which says, "Nettie Bongard." I converse with the piece of stone, telling her of miscellaneous things: the girl I'm dating, the latest in L.A., or how much she would adore my brother's kids. Then I weep, asking the same simple question, "Did your bust 'em up do well? Are you proud of him?" I hear the reaffirming yes come from a distant place. I kiss the slab, genuflect, and tell her I'll see her next year. Some things never change.

In the spring of 2012, as we pass the marble bust of Mark Twain, Heather Provost and I enter the banquet hall at the Lotus Club, a prestigious member's only club in the heart of Manhattan. A banner welcomes us as we make our way to a table. It reads: "The Stuttering Foundation Welcomes Converting Awareness Into Action Attendees." On the table, there is an array of nametags. As Heather and I give our names, the two warm receptionists welcome us and hand us our assigned tags. Entering the banquet hall, we are surrounded by stutterers and pathologists who have come together for one common goal—to support and find a cure for stutterers worldwide. Of the fifty people who have gathered in the room, I can discern who the stutterers are and who aren't. My fellow stutterers have the same look in their eyes that I see every day in the mirror. I am one of them. I'll always be one of them.

An hour later, I am called to the podium to receive my award for Converting Awareness Into Action. Jane Fraser, president of The Stuttering Foundation, graciously hands me the award. Instead of standing behind the podium, I make my way to the center of the room. I want to stay connected with those around me; we are brothers and sisters in arms. Unprepared, I let the words flow out from my soul, with no stammering or jarring, guttural sounds laced in my exchange. With ease, I express my everlasting thanks to everyone for such an honor, and then I say something I have never said out loud, but it is a thought that has remained with me since my early struggles.

"I am proud to be a stutterer because without it, I would not be the man I am today."

As I embrace their applause, a feeling of déjà vu hits me all at once. I flip through the rolodex of my memories. Suddenly, I am struck by the resemblance of my standing in front of a room full of people, as I wear a three-piece suit and speak words with elocution and fluidity. The situation parallels my recurring dreams as a child, where I am speaking to a large crowd and they are hanging onto my every word. The feeling overwhelms me, as my eyes turn misty.

Epilogue
Passing the Saber

Present Day

"D-D-D-D-o y-y-y-you th-th-th-think I-I-I-I c-c-c-c-can m-m-m-m-m-meet Yod-d-d-da?" Ben struggles to ask.

His voice echoes through my headset microphone. The audience is silent. No one moves. Ben looks around. He notices the confused look on the faces staring at him.

He knows.

Ben clings to his Yoda T-shit. He seems defeated by the critical glares pressing upon him. *Don't give into them, Ben.*

He wants to say something to me again. I can tell by his shaky body, his stomping of the feet, and his face contorting. I lower the headset from my cheek. My hand covers the microphone. This is our time—no one is invited.

As his little hand reaches out and tugs on my Jedi robe, Ben asks, "D-D-D-Do you th-th-th-think Y-Y-Y-Yod-d-d-da c-c-c-can help me t-t-t-talk l-l-l-like a J-J-J-Jedi?"

My eyes sting, and I feel the tears welling. No, I have to be strong for him. I have to be his Jedi. Better yet, I have to be his knight. I place my hand on his shoulder. I want to tell him something wise that I learned from my ventures, "Kid, you do it your way," "Life ain't cheap…a man has to suffer to get what he wants." "Don't try to impress anyone."

No, I must convey something he'll understand. I take a deep breath. I stare into his little brown eyes. "Master Yoda wants me to give you a message," I tell him, "and it is this…

Ben's eyes lock on me. His mouth drops. He is focused, as if he is hanging on my every word.

"My brave Ben, everything that is different in this world is judged with harsh eyes," I whisper as I point to the enormous crowd in front of us. "They will always look at you as different. But be proud of being different, for you are on a heroic journey...more heroic than anyone else here. That is why they'll never understand you. The hurt will come. The pain will come. The disappointment will come. But never stop trying to find your voice. Your voice is your own. Your voice is beautiful. It is your true gift. And when you search for your voice, you will learn something far more valuable...YOU. And soon you will become a warrior, a knight who fights for others in their pursuit to find their voice."

I unclip my light saber from my belt. I slip it into his delicate hands, "Yoda was expecting you, Ben, and he wants you to have this. It's a reminder to never stop fighting. Never stop learning. Never stop talking."

His hands tighten around the light saber. The light saber looks enormous in his tiny, frail hands. He stares at the gift like a winning trophy. A triumphant smile creases across his face. "Thank you so much," he says.

The four simple words spill out of his tiny mouth with no hesitation, and no stuttering. Wiping my cheek, I turn from the audience as I firmly hold onto the boy. I don't want to let go of Ben. I want to stay with him, guide him, and make sure he is okay tomorrow, and the next day, and the day after next, but I can't. He has the real world to contend with, and he must continue the journey by himself.

As Ben steps off the stage, Momma's words echo in my head; "Sometimes a man has to fight his own battles...alone."

An usher guides Ben to the side where he will learn his simple light saber combination. I focus on Ben's posture as he walks away. His shoulders are back. His head is held up high. He seems prouder, more confident. He walks as if he is ready to begin his arduous voyage, ready to take on the jeers, the taunts, and the dragons of self-doubt.

I place the microphone back on my cheek and exclaim to the audience, "Give Ben a round of applause as he continues his training!" The audience cheers for him.

I begin to clap as well, but for a different reason. I clap for Ben who has touched my life in more ways than he will ever fathom. I clap for the brave knight he will become. I clap for the little boy in me who is Ben, who is still battered, scarred, brave, and still searching for his voice.

I clap for both of us.

BOOK CLUB QUESTIONS

1. Do you think the main title of the book reflects the theme of the memoir? Do you agree that the book represents what its subtext claims, that it is an odyssey?

2. After reading *Voice*, do you feel as if you have a better understanding of stuttering and the trials a stutterer experiences?

3. What made the book memorable for you as a reader? What section stood out?

4. Since *The King's Speech*, stuttering has recently been thrown into the spotlight. What is it about this memoir that is different from other personal accounts on stuttering?

5. Because stuttering had a profound correlation with Damian's eating disorder, how do you think impediments or disadvantages in your life have led to other adversities?

6. The arts played a major role in Damian overcoming his impediment. How have the arts helped you prevail over your setbacks?

7. Whether you're a stutterer or a non-stutterer, what is it about the memoir that has inspired you?

8. What do you think made Damian internalize his imperfections to the point of solitude?

9. During his childhood, what do you think prevented Damian from being like Ross the Baker?

10. As he got older, do you think Damian mirrored Ross the Baker? How?

WHERE TO LEARN MORE

Websites:

Since they are such viable websites for stutterers, I will mention them once again. Whether you want to connect with other stutterers or you're trying to find a local pathologist, **The Stuttering Foundation** (www.stutteringhelp.org), and **The National Stutterer's Association** (www.nsastutter.org) have dependable information.

The Stuttering Foundation (TSF) website has informative material on how parents and teachers can interact with stutterers, how kids can learn dependable means on dealing with their impediment, and how notable celebrities overcame their stuttering. The articles and resources found on TSF's website are exceptional and worth viewing. Also TSF sends out three newsletters annually, so sign up on their website and become a recipient of their resourceful newsletters!

Social media:

Facebook: Even though Facebook is predominantly known as a place to reach out to old high school chums or long lost relatives, this popular site also contains personal accounts and educational material on stuttering. Just use search terms like "stuttering," "stutter," or "speech impediment," and you will be directed to pages that deal exclusively with stuttering. When you've found the page—what is also known as a "fan page"—click "Like" and you will get quotes, articles, and other valuable information sent directly to your news feed.

The Stuttering Foundation and **The National Stuttering Association** also have Facebook pages, so I implore you to find them, and click "Like" on their page.

You can also follow this memoir on Facebook by punching in "Voice: A Stutterer's Odyssey" in the Search bar,

Twitter: Twitter is also a resourceful tool that can put you in touch with information about stuttering. You can (hashtag) **#stuttering** or **#stutter** in the search bar to find other accounts that deal exclusively with stuttering. You can follow this memoir at **twitter.com**

/voicestuttersod, where you will find encouraging words and resourceful links.

<u>Search Engines:</u> Using search engines like Google and Bling, you can find a wealth of blogs that deal with stuttering. Type the keyword **"stuttering" "stutter,"** or **"stutterer blog,"** and you will be directed to an assorted list of blogs. Maybe you can start your own blog about daily hardships and triumphs. Who says you have nothing important to share with the world?

You can follow my blog at **www.branded-maverick.com/Voice** for updates on my daily experiences that you will relate with on a personal level.

Outside of Cyber City:
You can go to your local library or bookstore and find informative and personal accounts that deal with stuttering. Here is a list of possible books for you:

"Stutter" (Marc Shell, Harvard University Press, 2005)
"Stuttering" (Joseph Kalinowski, Ph.D & Tim Saltuklaroglu, Ph.D, Plural Publishing, 2006)
"Knotted Tongues" (Benson Bobrick, Kodansha America, Inc., 1996)
"Step Out on Nothing: How Faith and Family Helped Me Conquer Life's Challenges" (Byron Pitts, St. Martin's Press, 2009)

Acknowledgments

Before *The King's Speech* inspired millions of stutterers worldwide, the genesis of this book began as just a simple conversation between two doctors and myself over dinner in December of 2009. After briefly discussing my past struggles as a stutterer, Dr. Rachael Heller leaned over, grasped my hand, and said, "Scotty, you've got to write about this."

Stunned, I stared back at Rachael and her husband, Dr. Richard Heller. They unanimously agreed that my story would help those nameless heroes who couldn't say the words, and who were struggling to find their voice. In the words of the Hellers, "Write your story, and the extraordinary will come out of the ordinary."

That was almost four years ago. Since then, my mind, body, and soul have been dedicated to uprooting, rediscovering, and forgiving my past, which was as daunting and intimidating as any kind of psychoanalysis. Similar to how I found a solution to my stuttering, I had to hold the hands of those whom I trusted, and let their advice and honesty guide me through the difficulty in writing this book. With the help and humor of others so dear to me, I found my way through the labyrinth that comes with asking the poignant question, "How has stuttering made me into the man I am today?" Without the guidance of the following, I could never have completed this memoir.

To my publisher and editor, Lynn Price, who pushed me beyond my comfort zones to make this book the best possible manuscript. Her sharp and candid direction saved me from making too many wrong turns on this rollercoaster. Without Lynn, I would have never created the story I was meant to tell. Lynn, thank you for reminding me, as you so eloquently put it, "to dig deeper."

Behind every writer is a great literary agent, and Claire Gerus is no exception. Since our first conversation in December of 2011, I knew *Voice* was in the right hands. Her exemplary experience in writing has guided me in the past year and a half. Claire, thank you for elevating the book to new heights. Without your faith in this book, *Voice* would not be where it is today.

To my mentors and best-selling authors, Drs. Richard and Rachael Heller, I am forever grateful to you both for waking up the giant within me. Your constant tutelage has been nothing short of miraculous. You "rascals" have helped me formulate and organize my thoughts on a daily basis in what became the first draft of this memoir. Years later, your wise words still linger in the back of my head with every project I undertake.

To my manager and producer Heather Provost, for always collaborating with me and emboldening me to "write more."

For all those who took the time to read my manuscript during its early conception, you few, yet patient, souls, I am grateful for the most precious gift any human being can give to another...time.

To Jane Fraser and Greg Wilson of The Stuttering Foundation, thank you for all your encouragement, and for organizing a foundation that helps those voiceless stutterers find their fluency. Every day you create miracles.

Last, but certainly not least, to the two people who went through the confusion, doubt, and struggles that most parents of stutterers experience every day. They did the best that they could, and that was more than enough. To my Momma and Pop for their constant support in my recovery and their unparalleled sacrifices. My words are your words.